TRAUMA AND THE VOICE

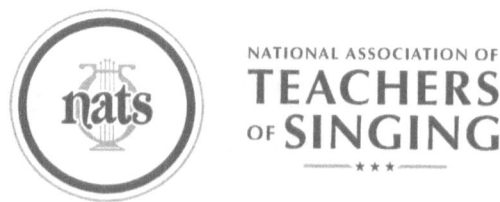

NATIONAL ASSOCIATION OF TEACHERS OF SINGING BOOKS

The National Association of Teachers of Singing (NATS) publishes high-quality books for singers, teachers, and other voice professionals. NATS books provide valuable and trusted resources that enhance singing pedagogy and support the important work of all singing professionals.

NATS is the leading professional organization devoted to the science and art of singing.

ABOUT THE NATIONAL ASSOCIATION OF TEACHERS OF SINGING

Founded in 1944, the National Association of Teachers of Singing (NATS) is the world's largest professional association of voice teachers and collaborative pianists with more than seven thousand members in the United States, Canada, and more than thirty-five other countries. Whether working in independent studios, community schools, elementary and secondary schools, higher education, or in the medical field, NATS members represent the diversity of today's music landscape, teaching in all musical styles. For more information, visit NATS.org.

RECENTLY PUBLISHED NATS BOOKS

Practical Vocal Acoustics: Pedagogic Applications for Teachers and Singers by Kenneth Bozeman

The Functional Unity of the Singing Voice, Second Edition Expanded by Barbara M. Doscher

Trauma and the Voice: A Guide for Singers, Teachers, and Other Practitioners edited by Emily Jaworski Koriath

TRAUMA AND THE VOICE
A Guide for Singers, Teachers, and Other Practitioners

Edited by Emily Jaworski Koriath

ROWMAN & LITTLEFIELD
Lanham • Boulder • New York • London

Published by Rowman & Littlefield
An imprint of The Rowman & Littlefield Publishing Group, Inc.
4501 Forbes Boulevard, Suite 200, Lanham, Maryland 20706
www.rowman.com

86-90 Paul Street, London EC2A 4NE

Copyright © 2023 by The National Association of Teachers of Singing

All rights reserved. No part of this book may be reproduced in any form or by any electronic or mechanical means, including information storage and retrieval systems, without written permission from the publisher, except by a reviewer who may quote passages in a review.

British Library Cataloguing in Publication Information Available

Library of Congress Cataloging-in-Publication Data

Names: Jaworski Koriath, Emily, 1979- editor.
Title: Trauma and the voice : a guide for singers, teachers, and other practitioners / edited by Emily Jaworski Koriath.
Description: Lanham : Rowman & Littlefield Publishers, 2023. | Series: National Association of Teachers of Singing books | Includes bibliographical references and index.
Identifiers: LCCN 2023016345 (print) | LCCN 2023016346 (ebook) | ISBN 9781538179451 (cloth) | ISBN 9781538179468 (paperback) | ISBN 9781538179475 (ebook)
Subjects: LCSH: Singing—Psychological aspects. | Singing—Physiological aspects. | Voice—Care and hygiene. | Psychic trauma—Patients—Rehabilitation.
Classification: LCC MT821 .T73 2023 (print) | LCC MT821 (ebook) | DDC 783/.043—dc23/eng/20230414
LC record available at https://lccn.loc.gov/2023016345
LC ebook record available at https://lccn.loc.gov/2023016346

Contents

Acknowledgments	ix
Introduction	xi
Preface	xv
Trauma and the Voice Teacher	xvii
Of Special Note to Performers: The Nervous System Onstage	xviii
What Am I Supposed to Do?	xx
Navigational Thoughts	xxi
Reading Guide	xxii

PART ONE: SCIENTIFIC FOUNDATIONS

1 Fundamentals of Trauma	3
Emily Jaworski Koriath	
The Truth in the Numbers	3
The Nervous System	8
Common Behavioral Symptoms of Trauma	13
Trauma and the Brain	18
What's Going On in There? The Brain's Response to Traumatic Stimuli	19
How Does Healing Occur?	25
2 The Polyvagal Theory and Voice Disorders	29
Heleen Grooten	
Stephen Porges's Polyvagal Theory Explained	32
Voice and Communication from a Polyvagal Perspective	35

The Impact of Trauma	38
A Case Study	39
Applications of the Polyvagal Theory in Practice	40
The Impact of Dysregulation on Voice and Other Complaints	40
Voice and Trauma	41
Body-Oriented Approach	42
Re-Regulating the Autonomic Nervous System	42
A Case Study to Illustrate the Effect of SSP	44
The Role of the Clinician	45

3 Attachment Theory and Developmental Trauma   49
Emily Jaworski Koriath

Attachment and Communication	50
Avoidant Attachment	53
Anxious Attachment	56
Disorganized Attachment	57

4 Current Research   63
Elisa Monti

Trauma and Functional Voice Disorders	65
Empirical Data on Trauma History and Non-Disordered Voices	66
Empirical Data on Diagnostics Criteria for Post-Traumatic Stress Disorder and Speech / Voice Indicators Utilizing Computational Models	67
Case Studies in Vocal Psychotherapy	68
Additional Related Methods	68
How Does This Inform Voice Teaching?	70

PART TWO: THE ROLE OF THE VOICE PRACTITIONER

5 Singing in Co-Harmony: An Introduction to Trauma-Informed Voice Care   75
Megan Durham

What Is Trauma?	77
Becca's Story	81
Trauma-Informed Practice	81
What Does "Trauma-Informed" Mean?	82
Singing in Co-Harmony	85
Embodying A Supportive Presence	87

6 Ethical Scope of Practice   93
Emily Jaworski Koriath

Transference and Countertransference	95
Joint Statement from NATS and VASTA	96

Survey of Teachers	98
Symposium at the National Center for Voice and Speech	98
Professional Ethics	100
Template for Student Disclosure	103
Professional Ethics and the Principles of Trauma Informed Practice	105
1. Safety	105
2. Trustworthiness and Transparency	107
Create a Culture of Exploration and Discovery	107
3. Peer Support	109
4. Collaboration and Mutuality	110
The Role of the Teacher in Emotional Skill Building	111
5. Empowerment, Voice, and Choice	112
6. Humility and Responsiveness to Cultural, Historical, and Gender Issues	114
Things We Can Ethically Do	114
Exploring Meta-Therapy (aka the "It" Factor)	118

7 When Music Makes the Wound   123
Emily Jaworski Koriath

Perfectionism	124
Shame	126
Mindset	129
Mindset at School	131
Feedback Skills	132
Paths to Trauma in the Studio	134
Race and Voice	136

PART THREE: A NEW WAY FORWARD

8 Finding Stable Ground   143
Emily Jaworski Koriath

Teachers and Stress	144
Signs You May Be Operating beyond Capacity	146
Sixteen Signs of Trauma Exposure Response	147
Just Don't Say "Self-Care"	148
Clear It Out	149
Creating a Trauma-Informed Culture	151
Secure Attachment Skills	152
Talk to Them	153
Listen	154
Attend to Ruptures	156
If the Teacher Has Avoidant Attachment	156
If the Teacher Has Ambivalent Attachment	157

9 Practical Tools and Best Practices   159
Emily Jaworski Koriath and Lauren A. Cook

    Two Existing Musical Frameworks: Social Emotional Learning and Trauma-Informed Choral Pedagogy   161
    Social Emotional Learning   161
    Trauma-Informed Choral Pedagogy   163
    Tools for Working with Attachment Adaptations   164
    Teaching Self-Compassion   168
    Self-Compassion in Action   172
    Consent in the Voice Studio by Lauren A. Cook   173
    Part One: What Is a Safe Space? Best Practices for Inclusivity and Consent   174
    Part Two: Our Bodies, Our Voices: Body Diversity as an Element of Inclusivity   179

10 An Exploration of Vocal Dignity   185
Megan Durham and Emma Lynn Abrams

    Opening Practice   187
    What Is "Dignity"?   187
    Voicework Practice   188
    When Dignity Is Denied   188
    Voicework Practice   193
    Honoring Difference   193
    Celebrating Choices   194
    Yes, No, Maybe Practice   195
    Centering Both/And   196
    Non-Dual Practice   196
    Re-Sounding Joy   197
    A Final Practice: Holding both Dignity and Humility   198

Conclusion: Trauma Awareness as a Social Justice Practice   201
Emily Jaworski Koriath

Bibliography   205

Index   207

About the Editor and Contributors   209

Acknowledgments

I REMEMBER THE MOMENT VERY CLEARLY: I was in my first apartment in Birmingham after an enormous life shift; I was reading bell hooks and Adrienne Maree Brown; I was in a coaching course with luminous goddess and Alexander Technique teacher Kate Conklin. Something happened and my body very clearly let me know that yes, I would write a book.

I didn't really know what it would be about but I started writing anyway, about the pain I experienced and that I see frequently in countless singers, and the ways that even well meaning teachers actually create harm in the name of building artists. I ended up creating a book vaguely about emotional intelligence and transforming the training of singers. By the time it was finished in the fall of 2020, I had also nearly completed my training in Somatic Experiencing and so I included a chapter on trauma. Many thanks to Megan Moores Haynes and Lynn Eustis for reading that early manuscript.

That book didn't get very far but Michael Tan at Rowman and Littlefield thought there was something there that he wasn't ready to give up on. Michael helped me to reimagine a book about trauma and the voice, something I thought I would only be ready to write about in a few more years.

I accepted the challenge and reached out to my colleagues in the Voice and Trauma Research Group. I solicited chapters based on each individual's interests and expertise. They in turn solicited further input from their network of colleagues and so we have a collective effort reflecting decades of experience and numerous tendrils of the trauma informed revolution.

I'm extremely grateful to the University of Alabama at Birmingham for new faculty grants which enabled me to pursue trauma studies and create this research identity; to my outstanding chair Patrick Evans for constant support and encouragement; to my colleague Edie Hapner who has already taught me so much (though I know we have miles and miles to go!); to Valerie Accetta, Lara Wilson, Elizabeth Fisher, and Cara Morantz who provide great feedback, professional mentorship both formal and informal, fabulous questions, and support when I need it the most; and to our libraries for helping me to hunt and gather materials from across disciplines. My work in Unitarian Universalism also taught me that values don't do much unless you live them, and I am profoundly grateful to Barb Greve, the late Elandria Williams, Susan Frederick Gray, Carey MacDonald, Linda Barnes, Joanna Lubkin, LeLaina Romero, Rebekah Savage, Sarah Jebian, and Bailey Whiteman for living their calls and inviting me to sit in my questions, examine the systems, and then to put my values in action. No one has modeled this for me more clearly and beautifully than my beloved friend Sarah Dan Jones, who loved me back to life when I was utterly lost, and whose life is both completely human and dedicated to lived ministry in every moment. I love you, Dan.

I wouldn't still be making music if it weren't for Lynn Eustis, Andre de Quadros, Dan Perkins, and Jonathan Santore who have all provided inspiration, mentorship, compassion in the face of many frustrations and tears, and sometimes a loving foot on the backside when called for.

It also turns out that writing a book is a very long and very challenging process, and I might not have kept going without the support and enthusiasm of my families (both the Jaworskis and the Koriaths). I come from musical and scholarly legacies on both sides and am proud to carry on those traditions. Most especially, we all owe a debt to my fabulous husband Tad who encouraged me, listened to me babble about problems with structure or new discoveries that got me fired up to continue and get this work into the world. He believes in me, so I believe in me.

Lastly, this work wouldn't exist at all if it weren't for the brave and brilliant spirits of my students past and present: from John Stark Regional High School, Plymouth State University, and UAB. Without you sharing your hearts and your gifts, I would not have seen the universality of these topics and the tiny sliver of our field where my deep passion meets a great collective need. Remember: art is a miracle, and it matters that you make it, no matter the form or scale.

Introduction

I FIRST ENCOUNTERED THE CONCEPT OF TRAUMA in Betsy Polatin's Alexander Technique class at Boston University. Like many wonderful teachers, it's Betsy's unique path that makes her work feel deeply authentic and meaningful. She was originally trained as a dancer, studied breathing mechanics with pioneer Carl Stough, and has also trained to become a Somatic Experiencing Practitioner (SEP). Somatic Experiencing (SE) is the trauma-healing modality created by psychotherapist and researcher Peter Levine, PhD.

I was studying the Alexander Technique in the hopes of finding more freedom in my body as I sang. I had been plagued by chronic tension since I began my vocal studies and was always interested in learning more about how bodies work and the ways that we sometimes interfere with their design and function. When I saw the word "trauma" in Betsy's book, *The Actor's Secret*, I knew that something new was taking root. If Alexander could give us the tools to notice our habits and make different choices about our use, could trauma healing get to the root of where some of these habits originated? And by healing them, could we get free for good?

I embarked on the multi-year training process to become a somatic experiencing practitioner myself, and as a result of that training and subsequent presentations at several conferences, I found my colleagues in the Voice and Trauma Research Group. We are voice teachers, singers, speech pathologists, and psychologists, and we meet monthly, and host zoom events to connect scholars in the field, especially since empirical studies in this area are still relatively few. We felt a calling to combine our work in these separate but related fields to create the resource you are holding now.

It's impossible to discuss trauma in the United States without acknowledging the centuries of harm created by the violent displacement of indigenous peoples, and the marginalization of those in Black- and brown-skinned bodies. As classical music and music education slowly begin to examine the influence of these systems of oppression, Megan Durham offers the following thoughts:

> [We] would like to acknowledge that many, if not most, mental health and somatically based trauma healing modalities in the United States are rooted in indigenous knowledge. Yoga, Buddhist meditation, Native American ceremony, and other non-Eurocentric traditions honor humanity's sacred interdependence with the earth and its diverse beings, and celebrate bodies as whole, innate sources of wisdom. In many cases, indigenous practices have been appropriated from their original intentions and deconstructed, decontextualized, and de-ritualized to appease a white-bodied, puritanical, patriarchal, and colonial lens. As we navigate our own biases, privileges, and shortcomings as mental health and voice care practitioners in light of this truth, we intend to continue learning, repairing, and recognizing the nonlinear, nonhierarchical journey of healing in all of its messy, emergent possibilities.
>
> A fundamental framework for decolonizing voice care asks that we consider which sources of learning and knowledge are currently valued. Voice professionals love to learn, gain knowledge, and make sense out of highly complex material. There is often a sense of accomplishment, control, and relief that comes with knowing which can be incredibly valuable; *and*, we can ask, what types of knowing are being prioritized, and whose knowledge is considered worthy?
>
> It can be useful to ask:
>
> - In my quest for knowing—whether cognitive understanding or bodily comprehension—am I also leaving room for mystery? Can I value wonder and numinosity as much as I value evidence?
> - Are my sources for knowledge consistently hierarchical, prioritizing the written word above all else? Are my evidence sources primarily from white bodies? What other types of knowing—spiritual, auditory, intuitive, embodied—are equally valid and perhaps underexplored?
> - AND: if evidence-based modalities have not been part of my experience, how might I become more aware of scientific inquiry and discovery, without feeling shame for how I have come into my current knowledge?
>
> If I cannot sit in not-knowing, am I fully living into the experience of being human? At what point am I trying to outwit my artistry, my creativity, my humanity?

*   *   *

Aside from the systemic issues that plague our institutions and industry, there is the incredibly vulnerable nature of the act of singing. It is so deeply personal to stand in front of anyone at all and make sound and be seen. Even for those without a profound history of trauma, thoughts of insignificance and doubt are rampant. Who am I to make these sounds? To take up space? To command this attention? Any attention? When a singer is also carrying a history of trauma, and their worth has been discounted by others, and they have never been seen or heard or valued, how does one even summon the courage necessary to have a lesson? How can you be present and stable in a room with one other person, attempting to be brave and show the inner workings of yourself? This is hard on so many levels because there's the act of singing itself, then there's also the fact that this person is usually standing before a gatekeeper of some kind, essentially asking to be validated. And there is so much fear. Will my teacher like me? Are they going to grade me and determine my future? How are these doubts and fears compounded when you have been victimized for being seen? The questions for teachers become: What do I need to consider as the person in the position of authority? Are my students safe to ask questions and assert their artistic independence?

As teachers, we must be honest about the potential for harm in our work. As bell hooks wrote in *Teaching to Transgress*, it is essential that teachers continue the ongoing work of self-actualization.[1] In healing ourselves, we become more able to hold the complexities that are inherent in our relationships with singers. She, hooks, goes on to say that

> [o]ur work is not merely to share information but to share in the intellectual and spiritual growth of our students. To teach in a manner that respects and cares for the souls of our students is essential if we are to provide the necessary conditions where learning can most deeply and intimately begin.[2]

Notes

1. bell hooks, *Teaching to Transgress* (Taylor & Francis, 2014), 15.
2. Ibid., 13.

Preface

TRAUMA IS CURRENTLY HAVING A CULTURAL MOMENT, but it is not a new phenomenon. The first studies of the link between trauma and psychological illnesses were created by French psychologist Pierre Janet at the end of the nineteenth century. Many of Janet's hypotheses were proven by developments in neuroscience in the 1970s and 1980s, but during his lifetime, his work was overshadowed by his contemporary Sigmund Freud's discoveries in psychoanalysis and was mostly forgotten.[1]

After Janet, significant contributions to our understanding of trauma were made by Abram Kardiner, an American psychiatrist who worked at the Bronx Veterans Home with World War I veterans from 1922 to 1925. In 1941, he published *The Traumatic Neuroses of War*, where he emphasized that war was not the only source of trauma. Kardiner's work became the foundation of the definition for posttraumatic stress disorder created by the American Psychiatric Association for inclusion in the *Diagnostic and Statistical Manual of Mental Disorders* (DSM-III) in 1980.[2]

In the late 1990s and early 2000s, when American service personnel began returning from tours of duty in Iraq and Afghanistan, both psychology and veteran support had evolved considerably, and the term *Post-Traumatic Stress Disorder* (PTSD) began to enter the public lexicon.

We have since come to learn that trauma is a fact of life. Over half of American seventeen-year-olds have experienced trauma or witnessed it firsthand.[3] The next person you meet is more likely to be carrying nervous system trauma (1 in 5) than they are to be left-handed (1 in 8).[4]

The criteria for PTSD changed considerably in the most recent version of the DSM, published in 2013. PTSD is no longer listed as an anxiety disorder, but has moved into an entirely new diagnostic category called "Trauma and Stressor-Related Disorders."[5] This classification encompasses eight different diagnostic codes, including reactive attachment disorder, prolonged grief disorder, and "Other Specified Trauma- and Stressor-Related Disorder (F43.8)," and "Unspecified Trauma- and Stressor-Related Disorder (F43.9)," which can be diagnosed when symptoms "cause clinically significant distress or impairment in social, occupational, or other important areas of functioning"[6] but the client does not meet the diagnostic threshold for PTSD.

The dense and specific language of the DSM serves psychology well, but the text is not innately relatable. While the full DSM entry will appear in chapter 1, we can start colloquially. My current working definition of trauma, paraphrased from Resmaa Menakem's book *My Grandmother's Hands*, is that it occurs in the body when your nervous system encounters more than it can process in real time. That "more" could be more light, more noise, more violence, more shame, or many other things. As we'll see in subsequent chapters, our in-the-moment response to this overwhelm is often a shutting down response, just as animals in the wild play dead. We numb out, feel like time loses meaning, and sometimes have no memory of the event, but scientific evidence reveals that while the mind fights to forget, the body remembers. The fight-or-flight energy that we were not able to actively deploy for survival in the moment remains in the body. Psychologist Peter Levine teaches that trauma is not in the event itself but in the nervous system's response to that trauma.

As voice professionals, we may be wondering what any of this has to do with us, but scholars and thought leaders in the world of voice science and applied pedagogy have already laid the foundation for this work. Recent scholarly texts have begun increasingly to include information about the ways that emotion impacts voice. Speech pathologist Leda Searce's 2016 text, the *Manual of Singing Voice Rehabilitation*, includes a ten-page chapter on "Supporting the Singer's Emotional Needs," and *The Musician's Mind*, Lynn Helding's investigation into neuroscience for singers concludes with "Emotion, Empathy, and the Unification of Art and Science." Perhaps the most direct conversation of the role of emotions in the applied studio is Paola Savvidou's 2021 volume *Teaching the Whole Musician: A Guide to Wellness in the Applied Studio*. Savvidou explores numerous body-based practices, including the Alexander Technique and Laban Movement Analysis, but also writes on "Mental Health Basics," including identification of some of the major stressors affecting students, and a brief overview of common mental health concerns including depression, anxiety, posttraumatic stress syndrome (PTSD), and panic disorders. What these examples make clear is that mental health is becoming less of a taboo among music professionals, and the field seems more willing to acknowledge that mental health does indeed play a role in both the learning process and the development of artistry. As we'll see in chapter 1, trauma not only affects mental health but also has measurable impact on the body.

Trauma and the Voice Teacher

The number one comment I hear from singing teachers when I discuss trauma is "I'm not a therapist." This is true, and it is crucial for each of us to consider our ethical scope of practice, as we'll discuss in detail in chapter 6. There are reminders of this throughout the text, as well as many ways to implement concepts from the research *within* the context of studio voice. Those who work with singers know that emotions and nervous system states are constantly present. Emotions play a crucial role in the learning of new skills and complex material[7] and in communicating that material to an audience through performance. When any human stands onstage or even sings in a lesson, their nervous system activates based on the fundamentals of human biology. Some teachers may feel intimidated by the idea that we are responsible for what happens to a person onstage, but, just like formants and optimal velopharyngeal opening, nervous system function is a scientific phenomenon that we can study, understand, and about which we can educate singers. So just like we need to know our voice science and our brain science, we need to be aware of the world of emotion and of trauma.

Some students will come to us having experienced what's called shock trauma or event trauma, tied to a very specific situation like a car accident, a surgery, an assault—a tangible moment they can point to. Some students will come to us with developmental trauma because of their upbringing or an event of which they might not even be aware. What I have also come to learn, as both a student of trauma and a person living with a very responsive nervous system, is that some of the things that are stored in my body as trauma are completely insignificant in other people's systems. I can't stress enough that this does not matter in the slightest. It is not up to us as voice practitioners to decide whether we think someone has been legitimately traumatized. If there is stuck energy in the nervous system, it's real trauma to that person. We all process things differently and depending on when things happen to us and what resources we have available at the time, seemingly insignificant events can end up being formative. It's also important to acknowledge that most students are likely not aware that they are carrying nervous system trauma. The teacher or clinician is not tasked with "finding" trauma and pointing it out to students or clients. Our responsibility is to be aware of the prevalence of trauma, and to adopt practices that contribute to nervous system care.

The effects of trauma are many and nuanced, but the primary problem for the teacher of music or theater is that the incomplete survival responses brought on by traumas large and small get stored in the body. The best singing and storytelling come from free and unrestrained bodies, functioning efficiently for peak performance. If there is emotional energy stored in the body, it inhibits a student's best performing, not only emotionally but physically and acoustically. It is inevitable that we will unintentionally encounter a student's trauma, whether or not they have the language to name it as such.

Of Special Note to Performers: The Nervous System Onstage

There is an important link to performance situations and how some performers seem unable to tolerate the extreme nervous system activation that occurs when one steps onstage. Under ideal circumstances, this should be regulated by our nervous systems as a safe level of excitement—while the physiological symptoms are the same as if we were running from a bear, to date I have never seen a bear in a studio class or recital hall. But some performers are unable to process this energy as "safe" because their fundamental sense of safety is muddled by past trauma. Practitioners need to know about this phenomenon because if we just tell a student to "buck up" or "get over it," we can be steamrolling existing trauma and reinforcing the belief that they are flawed, broken, or that something is wrong with them. I teach this in a neutral way, by providing details to all my students about how the brain, body, and nervous system react under fight-or-flight conditions. There are some students who are empowered by this information and can develop a healthy relationship to that adrenaline. Some students have found that, armed with biological knowledge, they are able to override an adrenaline spike through excellent preparation, or prevent it from happening through personal awareness and development of unique management strategies. Paradoxically, choosing not to fight against the rising energy can be enough to minimize its effects. We get into exhausting circumstances when we try to fight our own bodies. However, if someone has trauma in the system, this relatively safe set of circumstances could still feel life-threatening. Your body reacts the same way as it would (or has already done) during an active trauma response, so just the idea of being onstage and knowing that fight-or-flight will turn on could be horrifying. A student is not likely to know about their personal relationship to this activation until it happens, especially if they are not labeling past events as trauma. They may feel overwhelmed and terrified, or they will freeze. This is why some of them report blanking or blacking out. They remember nothing because they literally dissociate.

Dissociation is a trauma response where the nervous system gets so overwhelmed that the person goes numb or feels like they are watching themself from somewhere else in the room. Stephen Porges, the author of the polyvagal theory, explains that in situations of extreme duress, if we cannot flee, our body shuts down and reduces mobilization. As we'll discuss in detail in chapter 2, according to Porges's theory, when the vagus nerve is activated, it's a body-based response that sends a signal to your brain that something is not right.

Some mental health practitioners prescribe singing as a therapeutic intervention for clients with trauma, because the act of singing can stimulate the vagus nerve, creating biological harmony between the many systems with which the vagus interfaces. However, when our singing is fraught with muscle tension, perfectionism, and shame, we lose access to those healing benefits. Perhaps no one is more skeptical of the "healing power of singing" than someone who has been bullied, belittled, and shamed in their pursuit of vocal growth.

As a teacher, you never need to unearth the underlying issue for the student, and in truth, they don't either. What we're looking at is how each person's unique system is responding to the essential tasks of being a performer. Your responsibility as their teacher is to always be gentle and understanding when a student expresses terror at being onstage. Without even discussing trauma, it's important for teachers to normalize the body's response to the heightened state of performance because a student can learn to recognize this process as healthy and necessary and choose to cooperate with it for more freedom onstage. We don't need detailed storytelling about traumatic history. What's most useful is learning how the student reacted to the stimulus of being onstage under conditions of nervous system stress and how they have been operating since. That's where the intervention can occur. We need to ask singers good questions and then really listen to the answers. We work with people who are constantly moving in and out of states of fight, flight, and freeze, and we need to be able to guide them through that responsibly. We don't need to know where their reactions come from (and neither do they), but we need to be able to normalize what they are experiencing as healthy and adaptive nervous system functioning and help them learn to navigate in and out of that because *they are doing it anyway*. It's a required component of their training. As teachers in the arts, we are in the feelings business, and we have enough information now to recognize that we are also in the nervous system business. But up until now, we've collectively lacked the tools to effectively coach people through this.

We're biologically designed to perceive threats, and the nervous system has developed multitudes of stunningly different adaptations, each of which played an essential role in keeping you safe at some point. Whatever way your system reacts to overwhelm is normal. It is your system's innately brilliant and unique way of keeping you alive. Students must learn to recognize what is happening in their own bodies so they can ride the wave of that activation when it arises. I recently spoke with a colleague who was singing the role of Hansel in a performance when a panic attack developed that lasted for the entire second act of the opera. No one, not even her fellow actors or the conductor, knew that this was happening in real time. This is an extreme example of functional freeze: this artist and her nervous system were somehow able to finish the job despite legitimate biological distress.

We don't need to know students' stories and we don't need to heal their trauma. But we need to know that most students are carrying trauma—think of it as the rule and not the exception. We need to use that information to create studio environments that are supportive of healing. We need to talk about feelings freely and openly. We need to listen to our students and make space for them to think and explore in order to create a soothing or welcoming or safe or supportive space for their nervous system to process new information and learning and taking risks.

What Am I Supposed to Do?

Regulation is the term psychologists use for the healthy management of emotions. Human infants aren't born with the capacity to regulate their own emotions; we develop those skills in relation to the nervous systems around us. If we cry and people calm and comfort us, we learn that we can seek support from others and unpleasant feelings will pass. If someone responded to our cry with soothing words or presence, we learned to calm down or "down regulate." The calm, healthy presence of an adult helped our baby brains understand that our needs would be met when we were hungry, wet, or unhappy. Trauma practitioner and resilience expert Kathy Kain explains that this process is called co-regulation because the caregiver acts as an emotional role model and an external source of soothing when the child feels distressed.[8] Whatever emotional examples we see from our caregivers shape our ability (or inability) to learn to regulate on our own and process emotions on our own later in life.

Co-regulation is the most important thing that we have to offer to any human with a history of trauma or a highly sensitive nervous system. Harvard University's Center on the Developing Child suggests that "the single most common factor for children who develop resilience is at least one stable and committed relationship with a supportive parent, caregiver, or other adult."[9] One caring adult can help to repattern the brain after it's been disrupted by trauma.

The way that we show up with our students and clients is the most important tool we have. Therefore, the care and feeding of the practitioner is paramount. Your emotional well-being is a job requirement. This is another area where voice teachers' training differs greatly from mental health practitioners, who are usually required to be undergoing their own therapeutic process during training. It's only natural that working with others' emotions will spark activation in each of us. Learning how to process this in a safe and healthy manner should be required training for all educators.

Many of those who have devoted their lives to art take pride in claiming that music heals, but the unfortunate truth is that it doesn't always, most especially for Black, Indigenous, and people of color (BIPOC), trans and nonbinary students, those in fat bodies, singers with disabilities, chronic pain, or chronic illness, and neurodivergent students. While some thrive in traditional school structures, many have found that pursuing music in an academic setting hinders musical expression at a minimum, and can be outright abusive at worst. What do music educators need to become more aware of the prevalence of trauma in instructional practices? And what do healing professionals need to understand about how something that can be used as a therapeutic intervention can also be weaponized against voice users?

Navigational Thoughts

Intended Readership

This book is intended for the widest possible readership, including but not limited to the following:

- Singers and singing teachers who wish to understand more about what trauma is, how it functions in a body, and how it can sometimes limit or hinder artistic output
- Speech language pathologists who have a deep understanding of the mechanics of the voice, but want to know more about the singing voice specifically, the effects of trauma that they may see in patients, and why some patients don't seem to respond to standard treatment protocols
- Psychologists and other mental health professionals who work with singers or professional voice users

Terminology and Identity

When discussing cases, relating anecdotes, or generalizing the application of theory, we may refer to "clients," "singers," "performers," "voice users," or "singing bodies." These terms are interchangeable and represent any person who is seeking specialized care, or a greater understanding of voice use.

We will use they/them pronouns intentionally so that any reader may find themselves in the text. When relating client histories, all names have been changed to honor the confidentiality of the vocal workspace.

Contributing Authors

We are speech pathologists, psychologists, researchers, voice teachers, and trauma healers, in various combinations. You may find that some chapters seem to resonate with you more than others in terms of content: the first half of the book focuses on the scientific research that guides our understanding of the intersection of trauma and the voice, while the second half contains practical applications of the material. We encourage you to encounter each chapter with as much openness and curiosity as you can summon. The goal of this volume is to illuminate and encourage the pairing of the empirical and the embodied in service of healing and ongoing wellness. Because scientific studies in this field are relatively few, we disseminate the data that is available, we interpret psychological concepts based on what we know and see in practice, and use years of professional history to inform client care. Our hope is that wherever you fall on the spectrum, from rigidly data-driven to exclusively human-centered, that this volume can encourage each of us to take steps toward the liminal space where we all seek knowledge in service of our clients' highest good.

Reading Guide

Part One: Scientific Foundations

Chapter 1 provides an exploration of the physiological responses to trauma. What is trauma and how do nervous systems and bodies respond? To gain a deeper understanding of the effects of trauma, it is useful to start with the process of responding to threat and moving through phases of nervous system activation under ideal circumstances. By understanding the nervous system's circuitry, we are better able to understand chronic states of activation and the effects of unprocessed trauma.

In 1994, psychiatrist and neuroscientist Stephen Porges first published the polyvagal theory. The tenth cranial nerve, also called the vagus nerve (from the Latin *vagus*, which means wandering), is the longest nerve of the autonomic nervous system, and interfaces with the heart, lungs, and digestive tract. Of special note to voice practitioners is that the vagus nerve also branches into both the superior and recurrent laryngeal nerve, as well as muscles of the face and middle ear. Porges's theory suggests that in addition to the more commonly known nervous system states of "fight or flight" and "rest and digest," that there is a third component of nervous system function that he refers to as the "social engagement system."

Dutch speech pathologist Heleen Grooten has been working in the field of psychogenic speech disorders for over forty years, specializing in working with clients with "functional voice disorders," where no known deviation in laryngeal structure can be found. Her professional studies also led her to research directly with Porges, applying interventions based on the polyvagal theory to individuals with medically unexplained voice problems. In chapter 2, Grooten relates the fundamentals of the polyvagal theory and how it contributes to traumatic stress responses.

Chapter 3 provides an overview of human attachment theory and its application in the private studio. Attachment theory was first described by British psychiatrist and psychoanalyst John Bowlby in a series of papers published from 1958 onward. Bowlby's theory began with the basic premise that human infants need a relationship with at least one caregiver to foster social and emotional development. Further research by Mary Ainsworth in the 1960s and 1970s included the famous "strange situation" procedure, where mothers brought their infants into a room with toys, and the infants' behavior patterns were monitored as the mothers interacted with a stranger, left the room, and then returned. The theory continued to evolve and in the 1980s was expanded to include adult relationships. Current proponents of attachment theory teach that, based on our original relationship blueprint with our caregivers, each of us develop various attachment adaptations that govern all our relationships.

Part 1 concludes with psychologist Elisa Monti's review of current scientific studies relating to trauma and the voice that will by nature be out of date by the time this book is published. By attempting to codify the research that exists so far, we hope to provide fertile ground for researchers to connect to current data and design new studies to expand the knowledge of all in the field. Monti also includes brief descriptions of several existing evidence-based modalities for healing trauma.

Part Two: The Role of the Voice Practitioner

In part 2, we shift the focus from scientific study to practical application of the material. What does it mean to be a trauma-informed practitioner, and what adaptations can you make in client care considering the prevalence of nervous system trauma and our desire to provide healthy environments for vocal growth? Chapter 5 introduces the principles of creating a trauma-informed practice by Megan Durham. Chapter 6 provides in-depth discussion on the voice practitioner's ethical scope of practice as well as the differences between cultivating a supportive presence and crossing ethical boundaries into attempted psychotherapeutic care and includes discussion of the six elements of developing a trauma-informed approach as defined by the U.S. Centers for Disease Control. Chapter 7 is based on personal accounts from several singers about the unfortunate ways that vocal training has caused trauma or compounded existing trauma, highlighting historic and current practices that could be misconstrued by a student with a complex personal history. Our aim is not to throw stones at our colleagues past and present, but to provide inspiration with examples of human resilience, and to point toward best practices in a variety of settings.

Part Three: A New Way Forward

Part 3 brings all the data together to help teachers develop their own unique approach to trauma-informed voice work. Chapter 8 focuses on the practitioner's well-being, considering nervous system co-regulation as described by Stephen Porges, and in the building of secure attachment skills. Chapter 9 details numerous studio adaptations, including an essay on consent in the studio by onstage intimacy coordinator Lauren A. Cook.

In chapter 10, Megan Durham and Emma Lynn Abrams will provide their thoughts on vocal dignity: which voices are consistently heard and valued? Which are not? Through guided questions and an embodiment practice, readers are encouraged to consider expanding their approach to singing bodies and incorporating more intentionally inclusive practices. By each of us expanding our individual scope of practice to include nervous system care, we begin to collectively move the needle toward healing and to creating truly inclusive environments across every facet of voice care.

Finally, we'll conclude with consideration of trauma awareness as a social justice practice. How has nervous system trauma become so prevalent in the United States? Some potential answers may be found in the monumental study on Adverse Childhood Experiences (ACEs) conducted by the Centers for Disease Control and Kaiser Permanente. From 1995 to 1997, more than seventeen thousand adults completed a survey about experiences in their childhood homes, ranging from incidents of violence, emotional, physical, or sexual abuse, mental illness in the household, to emotional neglect. Almost two thirds of those surveyed had at least one ACE, and more than one in five reported three or more ACEs.[10] The lasting impacts of ACEs include, but are not limited to, higher rates of depression, anxiety, PTSD, higher rates of injury, and increased risk for both infectious and chronic diseases. As the number of ACEs increases, so does the risk for negative outcomes. The CDC has also outlined social determinants of health, or the ways in which we are affected by access to healthcare, healthy food, and opportunities for social, personal, and economic growth. We'll consider who is most likely to be carrying nervous system trauma and why, informed most notably by the work of Resmaa Menakem, author of *My Grandmother's Hands*, and Rupa Marya and Raj Patel, authors of 2022's *Inflamed: Deep Medicine and the Anatomy of Injustice*.

Notes

1. Bessel Van der Kolk, Nan Herron, and Ann Hostetler, "The History of Trauma in Psychology," *Psychiatric Clinics of North America* 17, no. 3 (September 1994): 584.
2. Ibid., 589.
3. Marc Brackett, *Permission to Feel: Unlocking the Power of Emotions to Help Our Kids, Ourselves, and Our Society Thrive* (New York: Celadon Books, 2019), 192.
4. "UN Study on Violence against Children," https://violenceagainstchildren.un.org/content/un-study-violence-against-children.
5. Anushka Pai, Alina M. Suris, and Carol S. North, "Posttraumatic Stress Disorder in the DSM-5: Controversy, Change, and Conceptual Considerations," *Behavioral* 7, no. 1 (2017): 7; https://doi.org/10.3390/bs7010007.
6. American Psychiatric Association, *Diagnostic and Statistical Manual of Mental Disorders: DSM-5* (Arlington, VA: American Psychiatric Association, 2013), F43.9.
7. Brackett, *Permission to Feel*, 27.
8. Kathy Kain and Stephen Terrell, *Nurturing Resilience: Helping Clients Move Forward from Developmental Trauma—An Integrative Somatic Approach* (North Atlantic Books, 2018), 20.
9. Ibid., 3.
10. "Fast Facts: Preventing Adverse Childhood Experiences," Centers for Disease Control and Prevention, https://www.cdc.gov/violenceprevention/aces/fastfact.html.

I
SCIENTIFIC FOUNDATIONS

1

Fundamentals of Trauma

Emily Jaworski Koriath

I've learned that when trauma is present, the first step in healing almost always involves educating people on what trauma is.

—Resmaa Menakem[1]

Trauma is a fact of life. It does not, however, have to be a life sentence.

—Peter Levine[2]

WHILE CULTURAL UNDERSTANDING AROUND TRAUMA has grown significantly in the past few decades, trauma studies are not at all new and date back to Pierre Janet's work in France in the early part of the twentieth century. The term "trauma" can be thrown around almost casually in social media posts and internet articles, but few people can articulate a clear definition about what trauma is and what it *does* in our bodies.

The Truth in the Numbers

Kaiser Permanente's monumental study on adverse childhood experiences (ACEs) shed tremendous light on the prevalence of abuse, violence, neglect, and other challenging circumstances in homes across the United States (more about ACEs in the preface and conclusion). It's important to note that since the publication of these findings, scholars have recognized several important qualifiers to the data: most of the study's participants were white, and they were interviewed in conjunction with other healthcare visits, which means that participants also had access to healthcare. Perhaps even more visceral are the statistics that researcher and professor of psychiatry Bessel van der Kolk uses to open the groundbreaking book *The Body Keeps the Score*. Originally published in 2014, *The Body Keeps the Score* spent over a hundred weeks on the *New York Times* best-seller list and has been translated into forty languages to date. It's worth noting that the following data were collected *before* the divisive election of 2016, the subsequent rise in hate crimes in the United States, the racial murders of Michael Brown, Tamir Rice, Eric Garner, Breonna Taylor, and George Floyd, among numerous others, and of course, the COVID-19 pandemic and its aftermath, through which many citizens around the world came face-to-face with the very real possibility of their own mortality. Subsequent research has begun to make the case that racism is its own adverse childhood experience.[3] Van der Kolk reported that research from the CDC revealed the following:

- One in five Americans was sexually molested as a child
- One in four was beaten by a parent to the point of a mark being left on their body
- One in three couples engages in physical violence
- 25 percent of Americans grew up with alcoholic relatives
- One in eight Americans witnessed their mother being beaten or hit[4]
- Twelve million women in the United States have been victims of rape
- Each year, 3 million children in the United States are reported as victims of child abuse and neglect[5]

Some readers may only associate trauma with reports of PTSD (posttraumatic stress disorder) in American military personnel, but as van der Kolk explains, "for every soldier who serves in a war zone abroad, there are ten children who are endangered in their own homes."[6] Confronted with such stunning statistics, readers will hopefully begin to appreciate the depth and breadth of the reach of trauma. But the costs are not only paid by those who have personally experienced these events. Van der Kolk goes on to explain that

> [t]rauma affects not only those who are directly exposed to it, but also those around them. Soldiers returning home from combat may frighten their families with their rages and emotional absence. The [spouses of those] who suffer from PTSD tend to become depressed, and the children of depressed [parents] are at risk of growing up insecure and anxious. Having been exposed to family violence as a child often makes it difficult to establish stable, trusting relationships as an adult.[7]

We'll explore the effects of trauma on relationships in chapters 3, 8, and 9.

Figure 1.1 is the verbose and somewhat overwhelming diagnostic language of trauma from the *Diagnostic and Statistical Manual of Mental Disorders*, version V (DSM-V), updated in 2013. It may be useful to consider the 1993 version of the DSM (DSM-III), in which trauma was broadly defined as "a stressful occurrence that is outside the range of usual human experience, and that would be markedly distressing to almost anyone." This definition went on to list the following unusual experiences: "serious threat to one's life or physical integrity; serious threat or harm to one's children, spouse, or other close relatives or friends; sudden destruction of one's home or community; seeing another person who is or has recently been seriously injured or killed as the result of an accident or physical violence."[8] In *Waking the Tiger*, psychologist Peter Levine provides a brief list of other common sources of trauma:[9]

- Fetal trauma (intrauterine)
- Birth trauma
- Loss of a parent or close family member
- Illness, high fevers, accidental poisoning
- Physical injuries, including falls and accidents
- Sexual, physical, and emotional abuse, including severe abandonment, or beatings
- Witnessing violence
- Natural disasters such as earthquakes, fires, and floods
- Certain medical and dental procedures
- Surgery, particularly tonsillectomies with ether; operations for ear problems and for so-called lazy eye
- Anesthesia
- Prolonged immobilization: the casting and splinting of young children's legs or torsos for various reasons (turned in feet, scoliosis)

Clinicians now understand that traumatic experiences fall broadly into two categories: shock trauma and developmental trauma. In shock trauma, we experience events that overwhelm our system's capacity to respond to threat in real time, such as the speed and danger of a car accident, violent attack, or a sudden fall. In contrast, developmental trauma refers to the long-term effects and psychological issues that result from abuse and/or inadequate care during critical periods of development. Levine explains that "[a]lthough the dynamics that produce them are different, cruelty and neglect can result in symptoms that are similar to and often intertwined with those of shock trauma."[10] In some cases, people who are carrying the effects of developmental trauma

Diagnostic Criteria (F43.10)
Posttraumatic Stress Disorder in Individuals Older Than 6 Years

- Exposure to actual or threatened death, serious injury, or sexual violence in one (or more) of the following ways:
  1. Directly experiencing the traumatic event(s).
  2. Witnessing, in person, the event(s) as it occurred to others.
  3. Learning that the traumatic event(s) occurred to a close family member or close friend. In cases of actual or threatened death of a family member or friend, the event(s) must have been violent or accidental.
  4. Experiencing repeated or extreme exposure to aversive details of the traumatic event(s) (e.g., first responders collecting human remains; police officers repeatedly exposed to details of child abuse).

- Presence of one (or more) of the following intrusion symptoms associated with the traumatic event(s), beginning after the traumatic event(s) occurred:
  1. Recurrent, involuntary, and intrusive distressing memories of the traumatic event(s).
  2. Recurrent distressing dreams in which the content and/or affect of the dream are related to the traumatic event(s).
  3. Dissociative reactions (e.g., flashbacks) in which the individual feels or acts as if the traumatic event(s) were recurring. (Such reactions may occur on a continuum, with the most extreme expression being a complete loss of awareness of present surroundings.)
  4. Intense or prolonged psychological distress at exposure to internal or external cues that symbolize or resemble an aspect of the traumatic event(s).
  5. Marked physiological reactions to internal or external cues that symbolize or resemble an aspect of the traumatic event(s).

- Persistent avoidance of stimuli associated with the traumatic event(s), beginning after the traumatic event(s) occurred, as evidenced by one or both of the following:
  1. Avoidance of or efforts to avoid distressing memories, thoughts, or feelings about or closely associated with the traumatic event(s).
  2. Avoidance of or efforts to avoid external reminders (people, places, conversations, activities, objects, situations) that arouse distressing memories, thoughts, or feelings about or closely associated with the traumatic event(s).

- Negative alterations in cognitions and mood associated with the traumatic event(s), beginning or worsening after the traumatic event(s) occurred, as evidenced by two (or more) of the following:
  1. Inability to remember an important aspect of the traumatic event(s) (typically due to dissociative amnesia and not to other factors such as head injury, alcohol, or drugs).
  2. Persistent and exaggerated negative beliefs or expectations about oneself, others, or the world (e.g., "I am bad," "No one can be trusted," "The world is completely dangerous," "My whole nervous system is permanently ruined").
  3. Persistent, distorted cognitions about the cause or consequences of the traumatic event(s) that lead the individual to blame himself/herself or others.
  4. Persistent negative emotional state (e.g., fear, horror, anger, guilt, or shame).
  5. Markedly diminished interest or participation in significant activities.
  6. Feelings of detachment or estrangement from others.
  7. Persistent inability to experience positive emotions (e.g., inability to experience happiness, satisfaction, or loving feelings).
- Marked alterations in arousal and reactivity associated with the traumatic event(s), beginning or worsening after the traumatic event(s) occurred, as evidenced by two (or more) of the following:
  1. Irritable behavior and angry outbursts (with little or no provocation) typically expressed as verbal or physical aggression toward people or objects.
  2. Reckless or self-destructive behavior.
  3. Hypervigilance.
  4. Exaggerated startle response.
  5. Problems with concentration.
  6. Sleep disturbance (e.g., difficulty falling or staying asleep or restless sleep).
- Duration of the disturbance (Criteria B, C, D, and E) is more than 1 month.
- The disturbance causes clinically significant distress or impairment in social, occupational, or other important areas of functioning.
- The disturbance is not attributable to the physiological effects of a substance (e.g., medication, alcohol) or another medical condition.

FIGURE 1.1
Diagnostic Criteria for PTSD from the DSM-V

are later subjected to shock trauma, which can lead to a compound trauma response that can be especially difficult to untangle. Colloquially, some writers have also begun to differentiate between what they call "Big T Trauma"—the life-altering events described above, and "little t trauma"—instances of cruelty, silencing, bullying, or shaming that leave their imprints on us.

Despite increasing clarity and understanding of the causes and effects of trauma, it can remain difficult to diagnose, or to pinpoint the exact source of a patient's distress. In part, this can be because the symptoms of either developmental or shock trauma are not always immediately apparent. As Levine explains,

> Symptoms can remain dormant, accumulating over years or even decades. Then, during a stressful period, or as the result of another incident, they can show up without warning. There may also be no indication of the original cause. Thus, a seemingly minor event can give rise to a sudden breakdown, similar to one that might be caused by a single catastrophic event.[11]

Another diagnostic curiosity is that each body seems to have its own threshold for which types of events are tolerable, and which result in trauma in the system. Even identical twins can live through the exact same circumstance, and one will experience the event as traumatic and the other may not. Some factors that contribute are the innate wiring of our systems: as we'll see below, each of us instinctively moves through phases of nervous system activation and chooses fight, flight, or freeze based on personal history, information available, and perceived levels of safety and/or threat. When a person has successfully protected themselves in the past, they may be predisposed to move through challenging events without storing the imprints of those events. Similarly, if we can notice the presence of something in the environment that could provide safety—a hiding place, a person who can provide care without harm—we may be able to weather the difficulty of our experience without it becoming stored in the body as trauma.[12]

The Nervous System

On a biological level, successfully navigating a traumatic event doesn't mean that we "win the fight" or eliminate the threat. Survival is the only measure of success, and the body will do everything in its power to ensure survival. Our reactions to perceived danger are determined solely by our instincts, and therefore it's not useful to attempt to place a value on one strategy over another. It doesn't matter if your system is predisposed to fight, flee, or freeze; if you survived, you won.

We'll discuss the nervous system in even greater detail in chapter 2, but we turn again to van der Kolk for a brief overview. He explains that the sympathetic nervous system (SNS) is responsible for the arousal of systems in the body, including our fight-or-flight response. When the SNS is activated, the adrenal glands release adrenaline, which speeds up our heart rate and increases blood pressure. Blood is also moved to the muscles to prepare for quick action.[13]

The partner to the SNS is the parasympathetic nervous system (PNS), which is commonly referred to as the branch responsible for human "rest and digest" responses. When the PNS is activated, the body releases acetylcholine, a neurotransmitter that can counteract the biological elements of arousal. Acetylcholine contributes to slowing down the heart rate, relaxing contracted muscles, and returning breathing to normal rates. The PNS is also primary in self-preservation functions like digestion and wound healing.[14]

Colloquially, we've come to refer to our survival strategies as "fight or flight," and with good reason. When an organism perceives threat, it may try to fight. If we know we are unlikely to win the fight, we will try to flee the danger if possible. But again, these choices are orchestrated by the body itself, and not decided at the cognitive level. Peter Levine reminds us that if the body perceives that neither fight nor flight will protect us, "there is another line of defense: immobility (freezing), which is just as universal and basic to survival. For inexplicable reasons, this defense strategy is rarely given equal billing in texts on biology and psychology. Yet, it is an equally viable survival strategy in threatening situations. In many situations, it is the best choice."[15]

Under ideal circumstances, the sympathetic and parasympathetic branches of the nervous system work together to help us detect threats in the environment, and then to return to biological homeostasis once we have determined that we are safe. Consider a relatively benign example from someone who spent fifteen years living in New England. You are outside for a pleasant but chilly walk, when you unknowingly step on a patch of ice that is hidden under snow. Your foot will slip on the ice, which may cause activation of the SNS: you may feel a flush of warmth; you may perceive that time is passing in slow motion; and/or you may call out or grab for something nearby to steady yourself. You slip but you don't fall, and if you stand still for a moment, you may be momentarily stunned; you may feel additional surges of heat or energy in the body, but eventually you'll catch your breath, maybe let out a big sigh, and look around to come back into the present moment. This is one example of optimal nervous system response: something unexpected occurs and the body immediately primes itself to organize a survival response. In an instant, your system recognizes that you haven't fallen and you're not in danger, and systems begin to return to normal function or "down-regulate."

In the 1941 publication *Traumatic Neuroses of War*, American psychiatrist Abram Kardiner was the first to publish the theory that the symptoms of trauma have their origin in the entire body's response to the survival event. As Levine went on to explain decades later, our traumatic responses are not actually caused by the originating event itself. Levine asserts that trauma is not in the event, but in our body's response to that event. He believes that ongoing symptoms "stem from the frozen residue of energy that has not been resolved and discharged; this residue remains trapped in the nervous system where it can wreak havoc on our bodies and systems."[16] Van der Kolk seems to concur, offering the following: "We have learned that trauma is not just an event that took place sometime in the past; it is also the imprint left by that experience on mind, brain, and body. This imprint has ongoing consequences for how the human organism manages to survive in the present."[17]

We'll dive into many of the physiological effects of trauma below, but Levine has also found through his therapeutic work that the body may sometimes retain survival gestures or actions that we weren't able to complete in real time. I had this experience myself when I was involved in a car accident several years ago. I was traveling down the street when a car pulled out of an intersection and struck the right side of my vehicle (sometimes called T-boning). This accident happened very quickly, and there's nothing I could have done to stop the impact of the oncoming vehicle, though I did see the driver pull out, and I remember realizing that I was about to be hit. Thankfully I was not seriously injured in the accident, but my body still has a strong response when I'm driving and I see a car approaching quickly from my right side. Even as I type and let myself think of an oncoming car, I feel a surge of heat, and the right side of my body begins to contract, right shoulder scrunching down toward my right hip, almost as if bracing for impact. I also notice that I very subtly start to twist toward my right side. If I let myself follow the instinct of that movement, I find that I want to extend my arms, palms up, almost as if I could stop the oncoming car with my hands. This certainly wouldn't have worked in the moment, but it was my body's instinctive response to that threat, and an action I was not able to complete in the moment to protect myself. During my training in somatic experiencing (SE), we watched video footage of Peter Levine interacting with a young veteran named Ray. Ray was suffering from terrible tics and involuntary twitching since returning home from combat. He did not have any such issue before his time in active duty. He had been to numerous doctors who could not get to the root of the issue. He was eventually diagnosed with Tourette's syndrome, but this did nothing to alleviate his suffering. Over many sessions, it was eventually revealed that Ray had stepped on an improvised explosive device (IED). The nature of these devices is that they are created to explode when they are stepped on. When Peter and Ray worked to follow the physical impulses behind each of the micromovements that were manifesting as tics, they were almost a textbook sequence of survival responses: turning one's head to determine the source of a sound, scanning the immediate area to look for other members of his unit that might have been in danger, and reaching for a weapon to defend himself. Ray was not able to complete any of these actions in real time because the device had already exploded, but their imprint remained in his body. Through a long therapeutic process, Ray was able to complete each of these survival responses and that led to the resolution of his physical distress.

These physical survival responses are one of the numerous reasons that many trauma therapists advocate for a body-based therapeutic approach. Van der Kolk has been working with victims of trauma since the 1970s and has been a pioneering researcher in numerous treatment modalities. He explains, "We have discovered that helping victims of trauma find the words to describe what has happened to them is profoundly meaningful, but usually it is not enough. The act of telling the story doesn't necessarily alter the automatic physical and hormonal responses of bodies that remain hypervigilant, prepared to be assaulted or violated at any time."[18] He goes on to stress that trauma results in a "fundamental reorganization" of the way our mind and brain work together to manage our perceptions of the environment around us. As we'll see in our discussion of trauma's impact on the brain, "[i]t changes not only how we think and what we think about, but also our very capacity to think."[19]

Integrative breathing therapist Jennifer Snowdon offers the following reflection on her experiences in trauma-informed practice:

> At the intersection of trauma and the voice we find the breath. Breathing patterns that are related to stress, anxiety, or trauma may include mouth-breathing, holding the breath after inhalation, restricting the movement of the diaphragm and lower thoracic region in favour of an upper thoracic breathing configuration, and rapid or shallow breathing. Our breathing is influenced by our nervous system state, based on what's happening around us now, as well as an historical state which may be alive in our bodies. Interestingly, breathing in these configurations can also trick the brain into believing that we are under threat, in turn signaling the autonomic nervous system into the sympathetic state.
>
> When we shift into a sympathetic state, our breathing changes to accommodate the probable impending action of fight or flight. However, when fight and flight do not come, and we find ourselves in freeze, fawn and other passive states, particularly when this is a repeated pattern over time, the breathing patterns can become habitual. Habitual stress breathing patterns can bring our bodies and nervous systems back in time to the moments when we were under threat, keeping the sympathetic state active.

All of these breathing patterns also might be found when one is singing. Singing, besides being a creation of sound, is a way to communicate to an audience. One might choose to utilize breath holding or upper chest breathing to communicate fright or sadness, for example. But what happens to the singer with a trauma history who is using these patterns in their singing? We have breathing that occurs with singing, and we have breathing that occurs with a sympathetically charged nervous system. We also have breathing patterns that we live with every day. Each day we breathe about 20,000 breaths, most of these without much attention to them, approximately one-third of them while asleep. With a history of traumatic stress, it is possible that the breathing patterns of everyday breathing will be those of mouth-breathing, upper thoracic breathing, and over-breathing, which would be classified as dysfunctional breathing patterns. Continuing to breathe this way, we remind the body to remain in its sympathetic state. Retraining the breathing to more functional patterns of nose-breathing, correct volumes of inhalation and exhalation, and lower thoracic configurations where the diaphragm and external intercostals are the primary drivers of breathing, can help stop the cycle of breathing patterns signaling stress.

When functional breathing patterns are established, and we have recognized the relationship between our stress breathing patterns and sympathetic responses, one might choose to use those breathing patterns in singing for artistic or dramatic effect, understanding the impacts they will have. We can uncouple our activity-specific breathing, singing, from our trauma histories, and from our normal, functional breathing when we understand and recognize these patterns in our own bodies. It should also be noted that although breathing in functional ways can lessen the triggers into a sympathetic state, retraining for functional breathing is not the only tool one needs when untangling trauma in the body and the unconscious self. It is also necessary to use tools of deeper therapy, movement, and other therapeutic methods to integrate past experiences.

Jennifer Snowdon, BCM, E-RYT, IBT

Throughout his career, van der Kolk and his team have researched the numerous physiological changes experienced in the body after trauma. He has discovered that one major area of disruption is in the body's production of stress hormones. First is the discovery that traumatized people continue to secrete large amounts of stress hormones long after the actual danger has passed,[20] not only in response to the original event but, as we'll see, when they experience traumatic recall; memories that are so invasive that they produce the same physiological reactions as if the event is occurring again in real time.

As discussed above in my ice example, adrenaline is mobilized to help us act in the face of danger, and under normal conditions, the body will increase stress hormones temporarily, and then those hormones will dissipate once we perceive that the threat is over. Van der Kolk explains that "the stress hormones of traumatized people, in contrast, take much longer to return to baseline and spike quickly and disproportionately in response to mildly stressful stimuli." The constant elevation of stress hormones can contribute to problems with attention and memory, and cause irritability and sleep disorders.[21]

Simply speaking, after experiencing trauma, our sympathetic and parasympathetic systems are no longer in sync. In ideal circumstances, these systems are constantly working together to keep us feeling safe and stable within our environments and ourselves, a state clinicians refer to as coherence. One measure of coherence is heart rate variability (HRV). We normally have steady fluctuations in our heart rate when we are at rest; the heart beats a little bit faster when we inhale, and a little bit slower when we exhale. But studies have shown that patients with PTSD have unusually low heart rate variability. Van der Kolk explains that this lack of fluctuation in heart rate has negative consequences on thinking and feeling, and on the body's ability to respond to stress. "Lack of coherence between breathing and heart rate makes people vulnerable to a variety of physical illnesses, such as heart disease and cancer, in addition to mental problems such as depression and PTSD."[22] He goes on to suggest that a biological inability to keep this system in balance provides an explanation for why traumatized individuals "are so vulnerable to over respond to relatively minor stresses: the biological systems that are meant to help us cope with the vagaries of life fail to meet the challenge."[23]

According to van der Kolk, "after trauma the world is experienced with a different nervous system. The survivor's energy now becomes focused on suppressing inner chaos, at the expense of spontaneous involvement in their life." This constant effort to control the numerous intrusive and painful reactions associated with trauma can eventually result in a host of physical symptoms such as chronic fatigue, fibromyalgia, and a range of other autoimmune diseases.[24]

Common Behavioral Symptoms of Trauma

In his book *Waking the Tiger*, Peter Levine provides an explanation of several common behavioral adaptations that result from traumatic experiences.

Hypervigilance

Hypervigilance is a constant sense of heightened alertness, or a predisposition to see relatively benign stimuli as threatening. Levine explains that hypervigilance especially affects the muscles of the head, neck, and eyes, as we are constantly on the lookout for danger. A person can remain perpetually primed to ward off danger, but this comes at a cost. When any change in circumstance is seen as a threat, we experience "diminished capacity to experience curiosity, pleasure, and the joy of life."[25] Immediately, the astute voice professional will recognize that tension in the head, neck, and eyes will have a negative effect on a free vocal sound, and a lack of curiosity might lead a singer to seek "the right answer" in music making, rather than becoming an active explorer of vocal sounds and colors, and the nuanced ways to interpret a poetic text.

Inability to Synthesize New Information

Humans have an innate orienting response that serves us well in our ongoing work of survival. We hear a sound, and we immediately begin to assess it: where did it come from? Which direction? What could have created this sound? We use the orienting response to categorize new information as safe or unsafe when we become aware of it. But when this response system is busy all the time because of chronic hypervigilance, any new information that isn't directly related to survival (say, fundamentals of vocal technique or nineteenth-century German poetry) leads to confusion and overload. Levine explains that "instead of being assimilated for future use, new information tends to stack up. It becomes disorganized and unusable."[26]

Chronic Helplessness

Chronic helplessness or "learned helplessness" is a condition where someone repeatedly encounters negative or uncontrollable circumstances and, in response, they stop making any effort to change the circumstances or their behavior. The term was first used in 1967 by American psychologists Martin Seligman and Steven Maier.

[Content Notice: I'm going to describe a scientific experiment that used dogs as test subjects. Feel free to skip the next paragraph if you'd rather not read these details.]

Maier and Seligman repeatedly administered painful electric shocks to dogs who were trapped in locked cages, creating a condition they called "inescapable shock." After the dogs had experienced several rounds of shocks, the researchers opened the doors of the cages and shocked the dogs again. A group of control dogs who hadn't experienced the shocks ran away as soon as their cages were opened, but the dogs who experienced inescapable shock made no attempt to get away. They just lay in their cages.

To a person on the outside of a difficult situation, it can sometimes be challenging to empathize with learned helplessness, but many traumatized people are prone to giving up any attempt at positive change. Van der Kolk explains that "rather than risk experimenting with new options they stay stuck in the fear they know.[27] "Levine offers another explanation: if your experience in the face of difficult circumstances has been to shut down or become immobile, you may believe that you lack the power to make any other choice. This belief is then reinforced every time you experience nervous system activation; you experience something new, but it immediately leads to freeze, shutdown, or overwhelm. It's easy to see how this cycle can become demoralizing.[28]

It's valuable for educators to consider the potential for learned helplessness in cohorts of students who have experienced years of schooling remotely due to the COVID-19 pandemic. I have seen this in my own studio, where both attendance and communication are slow to rebound to pre-pandemic levels, even though university operations are almost all the way back to "normal." Consider a student graduating high school in 2023: they have lived through a pandemic and its effects for three years, possibly including a year or more of remote schooling, diminished clubs and/or extracurricular activities, and limited social contact. It would logically be very challenging to stay engaged in school and fight one's way to graduation, let alone spend their last year with the additional tasks of researching schools, filling out applications, and participating in campus visits. If this student does manage to go through the admissions process and enroll in a higher education institution, it might be enormously difficult for them to consider taking risks, trying new things, or even thinking independently. Is it any wonder that a student might have doubts about their ability to learn the nuances of French diction?

Regarding students of voice, van der Kolk and his team have also learned that trauma affects the imagination, a quality he refers to as "absolutely critical to the quality of our lives." He attributes the failure of imagination and lack of mental flexibility to the constant pull of the past, and the fear that any intense experience or deep emotion will bring about the same results as their traumatic experience.[29]

Traumatic Coupling

"Coupling" describes the phenomenon where seemingly unrelated elements become inextricably linked in response to trauma.[30] Imagine, for example, that a specific song was playing on the radio when you were involved in a car accident. You may not have even been aware of this detail at the time, but days or weeks later, you may hear the song and have a visceral reaction or a traumatic flashback. A conductor colleague told me about a singer who needed to remove themselves from a particular performance because the score called for whispering. It turns out that this singer had experienced a traumatic event where their attacker whispered to them throughout their experience. Coupling dynamics can be difficult for both a survivor and a trauma-informed practitioner. For the survivor, many of these links may exist on an unconscious level until they are activated. Be on the lookout for language like "I have no idea why I am feeling so agitated right now," or even

"I'm freaking out" in response to a seemingly innocuous request. There's just no way for even the most experienced practitioner to anticipate a coupling that may exist for someone. While we'll dive more deeply into strategies of all kinds in part 2 of this book, one small adjustment in thinking is to take any response seriously, even if you can't see a logical reason why an arpeggio exercise might induce a panic attack.

Dissociation

Pierre Janet coined the term "dissociation" to describe the splitting off and isolation of memory imprints that he saw in patients.[31] In the simplest terms, dissociation describes a detachment from reality, usually because that reality is too painful or overwhelming in the moment. Some people describe periods of dissociation like out-of-body experiences, or like you are watching yourself from another point in the room like the corner or the ceiling. One of my trauma teachers explained this concept by telling us about a patient with an extremely stressful job in law enforcement who would get in the car, start driving, and not come back into contact with reality until after they had crossed the state line, having no idea how they got there, and no memory of their own actions. Some clinicians also describe this state as "functional freeze"; we are going through the motions but we're not mentally present, or aware of our surroundings. My teacher's client was perfectly capable of driving safely and obeying traffic laws, but their mind was somewhere else.

Many people's systems utilize dissociation as a way to deal with the pain and intensity of traumatic flashbacks. As we'll see when we discuss van der Kolk's brain research, traumatic memories produce the exact same responses in the body as when the events originally happened, meaning that individuals carrying trauma literally relive the experience over and over again. Dissociation can be the mind's escape from trauma, or dissociation can be the result of intrusive traumatic memory. If a person becomes so overwhelmed by the body's recall of the emotions, sounds, smells, and images of trauma, they may lose awareness of reality. These traumatic memories can overlap with the present moment. Van der Kolk describes working with a veteran who was immediately transported back to Vietnam any time he heard a crying baby.[32] As we discussed above, these memories will provoke the release of stress hormones, meaning that the loops of activation and dissociation will persist until the trauma is resolved. As van der Kolk explains,

> If elements of the trauma are replayed again and again, the accompanying stress hormones engrave those memories ever more deeply in the mind. Ordinary, day-to-day events become less and less compelling. Not being able to deeply take in what is going on around [us] makes it impossible to feel fully alive. It becomes

harder to feel the joys and aggravations of ordinary life, harder to concentrate on the tasks at hand.[33]

Physical Symptoms without Clear Cause

Through decades of experience and training, somatic experiencing practitioner (SEP) and bodyworker Kathy Kain has built a practice where she specializes in treating patients whom she refers to as "syndromal," people with complex medical histories and multiple diagnoses. Many of Kain's clients come to her to explore trauma healing after years of misdiagnosis, or frustration with the results of traditional medical interventions that "should" help alleviate their symptoms but don't. Kain often provides trauma healing in conjunction with a team of medical professionals already treating her clients.

In his work at the Trauma Research Foundation, van der Kolk has found that "somatic symptoms for which no clear physical basis can be found are ubiquitous in traumatized children and adults." These can include digestive problems, spastic colon, irritable bowel syndrome, chronic pain, fibromyalgia, migraines, chronic fatigue, and even some forms of asthma. In his work with children, he has discovered that traumatized children have fifty times the rate of asthma as their non-traumatized peers.[34] The team's research has also found that in patients with a history of incest, the proportion of immune cells in the body "that are ready to pounce is larger than normal. This makes the immune system oversensitive to threat, so that it is prone to mount a defense when none is needed, even when this means attacking the body's own cells."[35]

When our thoughts and bodies are overcome with responses to our trauma, we may work diligently to suppress our feelings and present an unaffected face to the world. But van der Kolk explains that this type of restriction takes an enormous amount of energy, leaving survivors feeling exhausted, bored, and/or shut down. The lives of many survivors come to revolve around constant bracing against threat or any unwanted experience, which leads to chronic muscle tension.[36] "Meanwhile, stress hormones keep flooding your body, leading to headaches, muscle aches, problems with your bowels or sexual functions—and irrational behaviors that may embarrass you and hurt the people around you."[37] In *The Body Keeps the Score*, he advocates for bodywork, massage, and various forms of movement to aid in the healing of trauma. As bodyworker Licia Sky explains in the book, "The body is physically restricted when emotions are bound up inside. People's shoulders tighten, their facial muscles tense. They spend enormous energy on holding back their tears—or any sound or movement that might betray their inner state. When the physical tension is released, the feelings can be released."[38]

Trauma and the Brain

The human brain is unique among the animal kingdom and is sometimes known as the "triune brain." On the most basic level, human brains consist of the reptilian brain (manager of instincts), the mammalian or limbic brain (the emotional center), and the human brain, or neocortex, where higher order thinking occurs.[39] Bessel van der Kolk was part of the first team of researchers to study brain scans in relation to traumatic events, and what follows is an exploration of what that research has shown. As van der Kolk explains,

> Research . . . has revealed that trauma produces actual physiological changes, including a recalibration of the brain's alarm system, an increase in stress hormone activity, and alterations in the system that filters relevant information from irrelevant. We now know that trauma compromises the brain area that communicates the physical, embodied feeling of being alive. These changes explain why traumatized individuals become hypervigilant to threat at the expense of spontaneously engaging in their day-to-day lives. They also help us understand why traumatized people so often keep repeating the same problems and have such trouble learning from mistakes. We now know that their behaviors are not the result of moral failings or signs of lack of willpower or bad character—they are caused by actual changes in the brain.[40]

The Human Brain from the Bottom to the Top

The Reptilian Brain

The reptilian brain is the most primitive part of our human brains, and it is already online from the moment of birth. Anatomically, the reptilian brain is situated in the brain stem, just above the place where the spinal cord enters the skull. This area of the brain is responsible for our most basic survival functions: breathing, our sleeping and waking cycles, feeling hunger, and then processing the food we eat and creating waste products, and notifying us of the sensation of pain. The body's energy levels are controlled by the brain stem and a structure in the brain called the hypothalamus. Together, these two structures coordinate the functions of heart and lungs, as well as the endocrine and immune systems of the body. We use the term "homeostasis" to describe the state where these basic internal systems are relatively well-balanced.[41] The reptilian brain also contains a cluster of cells known as the amygdala, sometimes referred to as the "fear center" of the brain. The amygdala determines whether a sound, image, or body sensation is perceived as a threat.[42]

The Limbic System

The limbic system is referred to as the mammalian brain because all species that live in groups and nurture their young possess this brain structure. As van der Kolk describes it, the limbic brain helps us to monitor danger and to judge what is and isn't important for survival. The limbic system is also the emotional center of the brain, and the command post for navigating our social interactions.[43]

The Neocortex

The neocortex is the top layer of the brain. Other mammals possess this same structure, but it is much thicker in humans. The bulk of our neocortex is made up of our frontal lobes, which begin to develop in the second year of life. The frontal lobes are "responsible for the qualities that make us unique within the animal kingdom. They enable us to use language and abstract thought." The frontal lobes are what make it possible for humans to absorb and integrate information and attach meaning to it, and to plan, reflect, and imagine.[44] Within the frontal lobes is the medial prefrontal cortex (MPFC), located just above your eyes. We'll come back to the MPFC below.[45]

What's Going On in There? The Brain's Response to Traumatic Stimuli

The Amygdala Goes on Alert

Sensory information is processed by the thalamus, which is inside the limbic system. It makes sense of all the information we receive and determines what is happening. It then sends that information down to the amygdala (in the reptilian brain) and up to the frontal lobes. The amygdala processes information faster than the frontal lobes do, which is why we refer to the fight/flight/freeze response as instinctive. It's the amygdala that decides whether the information we are receiving is a threat to our safety, not our rational brains. As van der Kolk explains, all of this happens "before we are consciously aware of the danger. By the time we realize what is happening, our body may already be on the move."[46]

As explained above, the amygdala is what triggers our survival response, including the release of our stress hormones, most notably cortisol and adrenaline, "which increase heart rate, blood pressure, and rate of breathing, preparing us to fight back or run away" says van der Kolk. Optimally, the body will return to homeostasis once the threat of immediate danger has passed. However, as van der Kolk describes it, trauma increases the risk that we will misinterpret whether given circumstances are dangerous or safe. When our normal cycle of activation and recovery is blocked, the body remains primed to defend itself, often resulting in agitation or prolonged states of arousal.[47] An additional study involved scanning patients' brains while they read a script about their trauma, prepared in collaboration with a mental health professional and a member of the research team. What this study showed is that the amygdala will react with alarm to the sights, sounds, images, and thoughts related to a patient's original experience even years after the event.[48]

What those early brain scans showed is that in cases of PTSD, the balance between the amygdala and the MPFC (within the frontal lobes) shifts dramatically, making it much more difficult to control emotions and impulses. In highly emotional states like anger, fear, and sadness, the brain regions that control emotions show increased activity, and simultaneously, various areas of the frontal lobe (especially the MPFC) show significantly reduced activity. What this means is that we lose access to the parts of our brain that help us inhibit our reactions. We "may startle in response to any loud sound, become enraged by small frustrations, or freeze" in response to human touch.[49]

In 1985, Kings College professor Jeffrey Gray presented research on the amygdala that showed that the sensitivity of this internal alarm system depended, at least in part, on the amount of the neurotransmitter serotonin available in the brain. "Animals with low serotonin levels were hyperreactive to stressful stimuli (like loud sounds) while higher levels of serotonin dampened their fear system, making them less likely to become aggressive or frozen in response to potential threats."[50] This discovery led additional research teams to experiment with a then-developing class of drugs known as selective serotonin reuptake inhibitors (SSRIs) to see if they could influence patients with PTSD (SSRIs are now a standard form of antidepressant). Van der Kolk reports that the drug did provide patients with a more reliable sense of perspective and helped them to gain control of these fear-based impulses, but he goes on to stress that "psychiatric medications have a serious downside, as they may deflect attention from dealing with the underlying issues" that contribute to a patient's distress.[51] While patients may experience relief of symptoms while on the medication, the traumatic memories that underlie these issues are not being addressed and will therefore persist.

The Thalamus Shuts Down

You'll recall that the thalamus is located within the limbic system and is where our brains make sense of the sensory information we perceive. MRIs conducted by van der Kolk's research team revealed that activity in the thalamus shuts down during traumatic memories. This breakdown of functioning explains why many survivors do not recall their trauma as a story with a beginning, middle, and an end. Because the thalamus is offline and not able to translate the sensory details of the event, it is stored as isolated sensory fragments: images, sounds, and physical sensations that are accompanied by intense emotions, usually terror and helplessness. The thalamus also acts as a filter or a gatekeeper, making it a vital component of attention, concentration, and learning, all of which are compromised in the face of trauma.[52]

As mentioned earlier in this chapter, no two people experience trauma in exactly the same way, and the research team had the unique experience of scanning the brains of a husband and wife who were in the same car during a terrifying road accident. While one spouse responded with the thalamus going offline as described above, the other responded to the study prompts by going completely numb. Their mind went blank, and nearly every area in their brain showed markedly decreased activity. Additionally, there were no measurable changes in heart rate or blood pressure.[53] The medical term for this reaction is *depersonalization,* an intense state of dissociation characterized by blank stares and "spacing out." Van der Kolk describes depersonalization as the physical manifestation of our biological freeze response. For traumatized people in this state, "with nearly every part of their brains tuned out, they obviously cannot think, feel deeply, remember, or make sense out of what is going on."[54]

Impact on Language

Speech pathologist Anna Rupert is the special projects manager at the Institute of Childhood Trauma and Attachment at the George Hull Centre for Children and Families in Toronto, Ontario. Based upon her work with the development of communication in children, she offers the following:

> Trauma has also been shown to impact language development, starting from even the earliest years of life. Through studies of children who have either experienced maltreatment or at an increased risk of having experienced maltreatment (e.g. by virtue of being in out of home care), research shows there is an inverse relationship between trauma and communication skills. Impacts have been shown most consistently in expressive language, receptive language and pragmatics (or social communication).[55]

I'm sure this is not surprising to learn given language development occurs primarily through the interactions with other people in the child's life, most importantly their primary caregivers. In the case of trauma occurring within the caregiving relationship in particular, it's not difficult to imagine there may be fewer language learning opportunities—both in the responsive interactions between child and caregiver and in terms of modeling and exposure.

In addition, when you consider the neurological impact of trauma and the subsequent suppression of higher-order brain structures necessary for language, learning, and use, language development can also be impacted by the fact that if a child spends more time in survival mode and their higher order brain structures are in shut down that's less time they're in a state of being that allows them to learn.

One reason why this may be of particular interest to the voice teacher is in the relationship between trauma and autobiographical memory. Autobiographical memory is part of what makes us who we are and how we understand the narrative of ourselves. It's made up of semantic memory, the memory of facts that we just know to be true, and episodic memory, the memory of experiences we remember. There has been shown to be a relationship between early childhood adversity and episodic memory; not only does this have an impact on memory functioning, but also the cohesiveness of personal narratives and an individual's self-concept.

Research has shown that those who have experienced complex trauma, particularly within the caregiving relationship have difficulty with recognizing emotions and linking emotions to contextual situations. People who have experienced neglect and other forms of maltreatment are less accurate at identifying positive emotions when looking at photographs of faces; they are poorer at recognizing sadness and quicker to recognize anger in ambiguous situations. This may be attributable to a heightened sense of threat detection as discussed above.[56] This may be useful information to bear in mind when a singer exhibits difficulty in comprehending poetic text. A person who has difficulty reading facial expressions or otherwise recognizing emotion in context may also misinterpret the state of the teacher or classmates, especially when the nervous system is activated and primed for threat.

Van der Kolk asserts that the team's most surprising finding during the brain scans "was a white spot in the left frontal lobe of the cortex, in a region called Broca's area. In this case the change in color meant that there was a significant decrease in that part of the brain." Broca's area is in our frontal cortex, above and behind our left eye, and plays a significant role in putting our thoughts into words. Broca's area interacts with the flow of sensory information in the brain, makes a plan for speaking, and passes that information along as movement instructions.[57] Broca's area is often affected in stroke patients when blood supply to the area is disrupted. The team discovered that Broca's area went offline whenever a traumatic flashback was triggered. Without a functioning Broca's area, a person will be unable to put their thoughts and feelings into words (another reason why some patients are not able to find relief through traditional talk therapy).[58]

Hemispheres Disconnect

The brain is generally divided into two halves, referred to as hemispheres. While the myth of our personalities being dominated by one hemisphere or the other have been debunked,[59] it remains true that certain functions of the brain are located in specific regions (like speech being controlled by Broca's area). Brain scans also revealed that during flashbacks, subjects' brains lit up with activity only on the right side. "Our scans clearly showed that images of past trauma activate the right hemisphere of the brain and deactivate the left[60] ... having one side or the other shut down, even temporarily ... is disabling."[61]

Loss of Self

Trauma treatment pioneer Ruth Lanius engaged in studies about what happens in the brains of traumatized people when they are *not* thinking about the past, and found that for the patients she studied, there was almost no activation of any of the self-sensing areas of the brain, meaning no sense of self-awareness, or sense of the self in relationship to the environment.[62] These findings can be especially relevant to the voice practitioner who works with their students to develop a sense of whole-body awareness. In a singing body carrying the effects of trauma, body awareness will be slow to develop, and may be nonexistent at first. For a singer with a lack of relationship to their own body, well-intentioned questions like "what does that feel like?" will become increasingly frustrating and isolating because the singer may not be able to feel anything at all. A subtle language shift is "what do you notice?" which invites a wider array of feedback.

Beyond the Best-Seller List

Trauma researchers and the public at large owe a debt of gratitude to Peter Levine and Bessel van der Kolk, who have been practicing in the field of trauma studies for decades, and who have distilled their findings into highly digestible material that almost anyone can read and understand. But to stop there is to neglect the fuller picture of research in the field, which is ongoing and continually evolving. Dr. Elisa Monti will present more on current research in chapter 4. Notably, researcher Nnamdi Pole conducted a meta-analysis of existing literature on the psychophysiology of PTSD. Pole selected studies in English ranging from 1980 (the year that PTSD formally became a psychiatric diagnosis) to 2004.[63] Pole reported that most commonly, studies included facial electromyography (or EMG, which was used to track muscle contractions), heart rate (HR; cardiac activity), skin conductance (SC; sweat gland activity), systolic blood pressure (SBP; the force of blood in the circulatory system when the heart contracts), and diastolic blood pressure (DBP; the force of blood in the circulatory system when the heart is at rest).

Pole summarized that in the studies analyzed, investigators measure the reactivity of body and brain in people with and without a diagnosis of PTSD as participants recall the details of their personal traumatic event. The most common study tool is a highly structured script-driven imagery procedure, individually tailored to each participant. The participant and investigator create a script of the event following a standard format, and when testing begins, the participant listens to the script they've created as it is read to them in the present tense. Participants are instructed to mentally relive the event while investigators measure their psychophysiological responses.

Pole's meta-analysis found that under the most stringent tests of significance, PTSD was reliably related to higher resting heart rate, larger heart rate responses to startling sounds, larger heart rate responses to standardized trauma cues (for example, combat veterans listen to combat sounds, motor vehicle accident survivors listen to sounds of traffic accidents, etc.), and larger facial muscle and heart rate responses to ideographic trauma cues (or the cues specifically derived from the participant's prepared script). Under less stringent tests, PTSD was also related to elevations in resting skin conductance and both systolic and diastolic blood pressure, greater eye blink and sweat gland activity to startling sounds, greater skin conductance responses to standardized trauma cues, and both greater skin conductance and diastolic blood pressure responses to idiographic trauma cues. Pole summarized that "in general, the idiographic trauma cue studies yielded the largest effect sizes across the broadest range of measures."[64]

The meta-analysis concluded that groups of patients with PTSD show higher resting heart rate and higher resting DBP than their study counterparts without PTSD, even though their SBPs are similar. The differences suggest that PTSD "exerts stronger effects on the resting phase of the cardiac cycle than the activation phase,"[65] which echoes evidence that suggests that the relationship between PTSD and heart rate may be primarily mediated by a reduction in parasympathetic activity, as opposed to an increase in sympathetic activity.[66] The quantitative review supports the notion that PTSD is associated with persistent hyperarousal, exaggerated responses to startling sounds, and elevated responses to trauma reminders. While the meta-analysis tracked results on all seventeen diagnostic symptoms of PTSD, results indicated that PTSD is most reliably characterized by abnormalities in the parasympathetic (or rest-and-digest) nervous system, and other biological systems that are involved in a person's ability to recover from stress.

Pole also noted two important gaps in the studies analyzed. First, the majority of studies published at the time of the meta-analysis were focused on middle-aged combat veterans, which means that it wasn't clear at the time if the collective results would generalize to different study populations, namely participants with different demographic characteristics and different trauma histories than those studied. Interestingly, Pole noted that the available studies did not examine the potential role of dissociation as a moderator of psychophysiological responses. As discussed above, many people exposed to trauma experience dissociation as a coping strategy, a "way out" when memories and symptoms become difficult to bear. Studies by Ruth Lanius and others suggest that patients with high levels of dissociation experience reduced reactivity when confronted with trauma reminders.

While an in-depth review of all current scientific literature is well beyond the scope of this book, curious readers may be interested in the writings and ongoing research of Wendy D'Andrea, Katie McLaughlin, Miriam van Mersbergen (who conducts the Voice Emotion and Cognition Laboratory at the University of Memphis), and Leah B. Helou, head of the Helou Laboratory for Vocal Systems Anatomy and Physiology at the University of Pittsburgh.

How Does Healing Occur?

An in-depth discussion of professional ethics and scope of practice begins in chapter 6, but as a preview, no singing teacher should attempt to engage in the healing of a student's trauma.

Within the findings of Ruth Lanius is a clue to healing: if trauma results in a profound loss of the sense of self, then one element of trauma recovery is to instill a sense of self-awareness. As van der Kolk notes, "The most important phrases in trauma therapy are "Notice that" and "What happens next?"[67]

Our ability to self-regulate depends on having access to sensations in the body, and this relationship does not develop overnight. Chapter 3 will introduce the concept of co-regulation, which is how human beings learn to take care of their own emotions. When we don't possess this capacity, we rely on what van der Kolk calls "external regulation—from medication, drugs like alcohol, constant reassurance, or compulsive compliance with the wishes of others."[68] This helps to explain some common singer behaviors, like seeking validation from the teacher, or becoming what some might see as the "ideal student," someone who hungrily accepts a teacher's every instruction without question. Even though the latter might sound appealing to some teachers, for the singer with a history of trauma this represents an outsourcing of creativity and thought, and perpetuates their dependence on others' opinions, rather than helping the singer become empowered and independent.

As a singer develops a relationship with their body, they are more able to track their sensations in real time, including those sensations related to traumatic memory or intense nervous system activation (such as the energy we experience in performance settings). With the help of a trained trauma healing practitioner, we must find ways of recognizing that all sensations pass. As we begin to notice our body's responses with a sense of awareness and detachment, we start to learn that we are strong enough to tolerate these waves of activation.

Notes

1. Menakem Resmaa, *My Grandmother's Hands: Racialized Trauma and the Pathway to Mending Our Hearts and Bodies* (Las Vegas, NV: Central Recovery Press, 2017), 13.
2. Peter A. Levine and Ann Frederick, *Waking the Tiger: Healing Trauma: The Innate Capacity to Transform Overwhelming Experiences* (Berkeley, CA: North Atlantic Books, 1997), 2.
3. Paul Lanier, "Racism Is an Adverse Childhood Experience (ACE)," UNC School of Social Work, July 2, 2020, https://jordaninstituteforfamilies.org/2020/racism-is-an-adverse-childhood-experience-ace/.
4. Van der Kolk, Bessel A. *The Body Keeps the Score: Brain Mind and Body in the Healing of Trauma* (New York, Penguin Books, 2015), 1.
5. Ibid., 20–21.
6. Ibid., 20–21.
7. Ibid., 1.
8. Levine, *Waking the Tiger*, 24.
9. Ibid., 53.
10. Ibid., 10–11.
11. Ibid., 45.
12. Ibid., 50–52.
13. Van der Kolk, *The Body Keeps the Score*, 79.
14. Ibid., 79.
15. Levine, *Waking the Tiger*, 95.
16. Ibid., 19.
17. Van der Kolk, *The Body Keeps the Score*, 21.
18. Ibid., 21.
19. Ibid., 21.
20. Ibid., 30.
21. Ibid., 46.
22. Ibid., 269.
23. Ibid., 269.
24. Ibid., 53.
25. Levine, *Waking the Tiger*, 156–57.
26. Ibid., 160.
27. Van der Kolk, *The Body Keeps the Score*, 29–30.
28. Levine, *Waking the Tiger*, 162.

29. Van der Kolk, *The Body Keeps the Score*, 17.
30. Levine, *Waking the Tiger*, 163.
31. Van der Kolk, *The Body Keeps the* Score, 182.
32. Ibid., 66.
33. Ibid., 67.
34. Ibid., 100.
35. Ibid., 129.
36. Ibid., 267.
37. Ibid., 235.
38. Ibid., 218–19.
39. Levine, *Waking the Tiger*, 17.
40. Van der Kolk, *The Body Keeps the Score*, 3.
41. Ibid., 56.
42. Ibid., 33.
43. Ibid., 56.
44. Ibid., 58.
45. Ibid., 62.
46. Ibid., 60–61.
47. Ibid., 61–62.
48. Ibid., 42.
49. Ibid., 62–63.
50. Ibid., 33.
51. Ibid., 36–37.
52. Ibid., 70.
53. Ibid., 71.
54. Ibid., 72.
55. Allen and Oliver, 1982; Coster et al., 1989; Beeghly and Cicchetti, 1994; Eigsti and Cicchetti, 2004; Fox et al., 1988.
56. Research summarized by Ashley Brien, Tiffany L. Hutchins, Carol Westby, "Autobiographical Memory in Autism Spectrum Disorder, Attention-Deficit / Hyperactivity Disorder, Hearing Loss, and Childhood Trauma: Implications for Social Communication Intervention," *Language, Speech and Hearing Services in Schools* 52, no. 1 (January 19, 2021): 39–59.
57. "Broca's Area Is the Brain's Scriptwriter, Shaping Speech, Study Finds," Johns Hopkins Medicine, February 17, 2015, https://www.hopkinsmedicine.org/news/media/releases/brocas_area_is_the_brains_scriptwriter_shaping_speech_study_finds (accessed December 12, 2022).
58. Van der Kolk, *The Body Keeps the Score*, 43.
59. Robert H. Shmerling, "Right Brain / Left Brain, Right?" Harvard Health Publishing, March 4, 2022, https://www.health.harvard.edu/blog/right-brainleft-brain-right-2017082512222 (accessed December 22, 2022).
60. Van der Kolk, *The Body Keeps the* Score, 44.
61. Ibid., 45.
62. Ibid., 92.

63. Nnamdi Pole, "The Psychophysiology of Posttraumatic Stress Disorder: A Meta-Analysis." *Psychological Bulletin* vol. 133, no. 5 (2007): 725–46. doi:10.1037/0033-2909.133.5.725.

64. Ibid., 740.

65. Pole, "The Psychophysiology of Posttraumatic Stress Disorder," 726.

66. Ibid.

67. Van der Kolk, *The Body Keeps the Score*, 99.

68. Ibid.

2

The Polyvagal Theory and Voice Disorders

Heleen Grooten

IN 1994 PSYCHIATRIST[1] AND NEUROSCIENTIST Stephen Porges first published the polyvagal theory. The tenth cranial nerve, also called the vagus nerve (from the Latin *vagus*, which means wandering), is the longest nerve of the autonomic nervous system, and interfaces with the heart, lungs, and digestive tract. Of special note to voice practitioners is that the vagus nerve also branches into both the superior and recurrent laryngeal nerve, as well as muscles of the face and the middle ear. In other words, every system of the body required for singing is connected to the vagus nerve. Porges's theory suggests that in addition to the more commonly known nervous system states of "fight or flight" and "rest and digest," that there is a third component of nervous system function that he refers to as the "social engagement system."[2] But before we discuss the intricacies of the polyvagal theory, it may be useful to review standard procedures of voice care so we can more closely understand how Porges's work relates to the treatment of voice disorders, and our understanding of the effects of trauma on the voice from a nervous system perspective. The following is in no way comprehensive; a complete consideration of voice disorders from a medical perspective is outside the scope of this book, and many extraordinary resources exist.

[editor's note: Heleen Grooten practices speech pathology in The Netherlands. Terms and roles may not align directly with medical systems in all countries. This chapter has been translated from Dutch]

Signs of a voice disorder include sudden but lingering changes in pitch, volume, tone, or overall vocal quality. If a singer in your studio presents with persistent vocal issues for more than two weeks, refer them to their primary care doctor or general practitioner for an overall wellness check. If there is no obvious explanation for their symptoms (such as asthma, allergies, or bronchitis), often the first course of recommended action is voice rest and increased hydration. If symptoms persist after this initial intervention, the voice user will then be referred to an otolaryngologist, more commonly referred to as an ear, nose, and throat doctor (ENT) to investigate whether a physical abnormality is involved. In the European medical system, this professional is known as a phoniatrician. The ENT examines the larynx, throat, and nose with a laryngoscope (a small, flexible camera that is inserted into a nostril) in order to visually examine the vocal mechanism and look for structural issues.

There are a number of natural causes of voice disorders, including tissue growths such as nodules or other lesions, inflammation and swelling, nerve problems, biological irregularity, and hormones. For example, a congenital abnormality in the larynx may result in the vocal folds not closing together properly, so that not all the exhaled air is converted into sound and therefore the voice user becomes hoarse. These conditions are called *organic abnormalities* or *organic voice disorders*.[3]

Anyone who uses the voice intensively due to their profession, such as a classroom teacher, actor, or customer service agent is clinically referred to as a professional voice user. Long, loud, overly tense, or otherwise inefficient use of the voice can cause a lump, irritation, or inflammation to one or both vocal folds. This group of complaints is called *functional abnormalities* or *functional disorders*:[4] the abnormality is caused by the way the client uses their voice. Common symptoms of abnormalities in the larynx are hoarseness, fatigue during speaking and or singing, and often lack of volume; a client can't produce louder sounds and they have a hard time being understood by others. In spite of these symptoms, the client's vocal mechanism will appear normal when viewed by the laryngoscope.

A *psychogenic voice disorder*[5] has no apparent physical cause and occurs when psychological stressors lead to habitual, maladaptive speaking habits. Common symptoms in a client with a psychogenic disorder are a strained or raspy voice, lack of volume, and sometimes a complete loss of voice. The American Speech-Language-Hearing Association (ASHA) acknowledges that chronic stress, depression, and anxiety can all contribute to psychogenic voice disorders. It is important for voice teachers to understand that, in the medical world, psychological trauma and other emotional states are valid causes of vocal irregularity. For speech pathologists, when a psychogenic disorder is suspected, clients are referred to a psychologist or psychiatrist for additional examination and addressing the root psychological concern is the key to resolution of the disorder. While some singing teachers and university administrators resist acknowledging that students' emotional lives influence their singing, the medical community acknowledges and embraces this truth in the service of vocal health.

After a physical examination by an ENT, a speech therapist often comes into the picture. In a number of clinical settings, a speech therapist supports the ENT in examining and diagnosing the complaint and can collaborate in order to find out to what extent a better voice can be induced.

In my forty-three years as a speech therapist, I have specialized in the treatment of people with voice disorders. The speech therapist can treat a whole spectrum of disorders such as stuttering and language/speech development disorders, hearing and audiation issues, or swallowing disorders, but my interest from the beginning of my training was the field of voice and voice disorders.

Immediately after my graduation, I started a practice for voice disorders, as there was a great need for speech therapists with a feel for voice. I started my practice in the farmhouse in the woods that my husband and I shared. Clients came from far and wide for treatment on referral from one particular doctor.

I treated many clients successfully with breathing and voice exercises and often noticed that there was also a "story" playing in the background of the complaint, which seemed to underlie their voice problem. Only later did I understand that all these clients were referred to me by this doctor because he suspected that there was a psychological cause in the background of the voice disorder. The combination of these factors has led to a lifelong search for an explanation of the origin of these complaints. I regularly saw that in many cases, technical exercises only brought temporary relief, even though the client faithfully did the work. A listening ear, breathing exercises, and a walk in the woods near the practice before or after the session seemed to have an important regulating function.

In recent years, the term medically unexplained symptoms (MUS), has also attracted attention. Research has shown that medical specialists are unable to interpret or resolve 40 to 60 percent of the symptoms patients present to them.[6] That confirmed my impression: functional voice disorders are not always based on "incorrect voice use," as seen in speech therapy. People with MUS are often referred simultaneously to various medical specialists for testing, and also look for their own answers to their health questions in the realm of alternative medicine. This is not only costly for the patient but can also yield additional trauma as they put their faith in source after source, only to have their hopes for answers and resolution repeatedly dashed.

Out of personal and professional interest, I followed a two-year training in systemic constellations in the year 2000. This is the work of German psychotherapist Bert Hellinger,[7] who introduced constellations as a way to "reveal and transform" the many patterns at work in family systems. This brought me the insight that in many families there are strongly disrupting patterns, which can have a great impact on clients and their psychological and physical well-being.

An international study of "misunderstood complaints" initiated by the German psychiatrist Weber and involving teams from seven different countries in Europe and South America, showed that complaints and symptoms can have an origin in families. If these patterns are brought to light, it can bring about a miraculous change both in the system and in the specific complaint.[8]

After my training in systemic constellations, I started training in somatic experiencing,[9] a three-year body-oriented trauma therapy training. This is an intensive training, with many hours of supervision and learning therapy, which enabled me to understand and process many of my own patterns. I also learned about the role of the autonomic nervous system (ANS) and the vagus nerve in trauma. My personal interest in this topic led me to the polyvagal theory (PVT) and Dr. Stephen Porges, its founder. Although as a speech therapist I knew that this cranial nerve innervates the larynx and vocal folds, it only then became clear to me that this longest cranial nerve also controls, for example, the intestines and the heart. I suddenly understood that many other complaints that my clients reported were complaints of one system.

Contact with Dr. Porges and his scientific collaborators has led to research, new insights, and the implementation of the theory and method in my work and that of others. Clients feel empowered by knowledge about the ANS that is passed on to them in conjunction with the treatment of their "misunderstood complaints." They see how the dysregulation of their autonomic nervous system could have arisen from what they experienced in their families and/or their own lives and how they can learn to regulate themselves again. As a result, their complaints may disappear or be greatly reduced. They see that talking a lot about what they have experienced does not necessarily contribute to essential recovery and that a body-oriented, nonjudgmental approach brings them recovery.

Stephen Porges's Polyvagal Theory Explained

The polyvagal theory makes a vital contribution to understanding the ANS and its many functions. The ANS is a system formed during evolution that focuses on survival. You'll recall from chapter 1 that there is a regulatory, resting part called the parasympathetic and an activating part called the sympathetic. The vagus nerve, the longest cranial nerve and the namesake of the PVT is a parasympathetic nerve. The ANS operates unconsciously, outside of our cognition. Explained another way, the ANS perceives threat or safety *first*, and then communicates those states from the body to the brain in order to elicit action. Evolutionarily ancient parts of the brain and nervous system still exist in humans, though newer brain processes have evolved over millennia in response to our changing environments. The oldest part of the parasympathetic is the basis of our ANS and is controlled by a branch of the vagus called dorsal vagus.[10] This branch, like other cranial nerves, originates in the brainstem. Its function is to control the organs below the diaphragm. In cases of threat, primitive animal species survive by withdrawing, keeping quiet, not making a sound, and setting their digestion to the economy burner. These primitive patterns can also occur in humans as a survival response in the face of mortal danger. From these primitive animals, the sympathetic system has evolved, the activating part of the ANS. It is formed by a group of fibers of the spinal cord system, which runs along the length of the spine from the first thoracic vertebra (T1) to the second lumbar vertebra (L2). At rest, the sympathetic system takes care of the organs above the diaphragm, such as the heart and lungs.[11] If, in the face of danger, action is required, the sympathetic branch of the nervous system enables a fight-or-flight response; it can accelerate breath and heart rate in tenths of seconds and build muscle tension. It enables rapid scanning of the outside world using the senses.

Mammals, including humans, have a third way to get to safety: by connecting with other members of their species. Together with four other cranial nerves (the fifth, seventh, ninth, and eleventh cranial nerves), the vagus (the tenth cranial nerve) forms what Porges calls the social engagement system,[12] also called the ventral vagal complex. Together, these cranial nerves are responsible for social engagement and interaction with peers through the eyes, ears, larynx, throat, heart, and lungs. The social engagement system enables humans to communicate, form friendships, care for others, and engage in social activities such as eating and drinking together. The vagus branch involved in the social engagement system is called the ventral vagus.

Stage One: *Ventral Vagal (Social Engagement)*	We are able to safely communicate with others and also engage in self-soothing. We may attempt to talk our way out of a conflict or engage cognitively to attempt to solve the problem. We may notice sympathetic activation (for example, sweating or shortness of breath), but those biological responses are manageable.
Stage Two: *Sympathetic Activation (Mobilization)*	If we can't get our needs met while we're in our social engagement system, the sympathetic nervous system will activate, producing adrenaline in conjunction with our instincts to fight or flee. There is muscle tension in the jaw, neck and shoulders, heart rate accelerates, and breathing is high and fast.
Stage Three: *Dorsal Vagal (Immobilization)*	When all else fails, the body begins to conserve oxygen, decrease the heart rate and respiration, and lowers the use of energy to slow down and shut down the body. There is minimal movement and metabolism.

FIGURE 2.1
Hierarchy of Nervous System Response as Proposed by Stephen Porges

Porges formulated the polyvagal theory to explain the interaction between the dorsal and ventral vagus and the sympathetic nervous system, and his theory states that there is a clear hierarchy of nervous system states; he hypothesizes that activation of these states runs in a sequence, based on brain evolution.[13] When there is safety and social connection, all three systems are in balance with each other. In safety, the ventral vagus is active, and if a threat appears and the body deems it to be insignificant, it's the ventral vagal system that keeps the sympathetic system from taking over.

If the body decides that mobilization is necessary, we can defend ourselves by moving into sympathetic activation. As discussed in chapter 1, the body prepares to fight or flee by secreting adrenaline, accelerating the heartbeat, and priming the muscles for action. In the case of a prolonged sympathetic survival response, functions such as swallowing, chewing, eating, drinking, and voice use may be disrupted.[14] There is tension in the face, the eye muscles are often pinched, and there may be continuous tightening of the jaw. The heart rate is greatly increased or irregular, blood pressure is elevated, and breathing is rapid and clavicular. Our hearing is focused on outside sounds,[15] especially what some clinicians refer to as "predator sounds," or the extreme ends of both high and low frequency. Human voices are therefore less understood. If this state persists for a long time, hypersensitivity to sound can occur.[16] When we're in this state, we will also present with hyperarousal; we are easily irritated, speak loudly and quickly, or startle easily. It will take some time, but when the threat has passed, we ease our way back to the calm provided by the ventral vagus.

If a situation is so threatening that activity of the dorsal vagus is necessary, we automatically withdraw and cannot make contact with others. The immobility brought on by the dorsal vagal is designed to be time-limited; under normal biological conditions, when the threat passes and the body perceives safety, we slowly emerge from the dorsal vagal state and can return to feeling safe when interacting with others. In other words, when people have a dorsal vagal reaction, they can be co-regulated by a safe person in their environment and return to a ventral vagal state. However, a period of prolonged stress can bring about a state of chronic dysregulation. When there is a chronic life-threatening situation, the ANS is left with one last survival response: dorsal shutdown. Everything that costs energy is automatically and unconsciously avoided. This has an impact on vital functions such as heart rate, breathing, and digestion: the heart rate slows down and breathing becomes slower and shallower. The mental state is characterized by "absence" (clinically referred to as *dissociation*), others may faint. People become silent and might even have no voice at all (aphonia) and may develop problems with word finding and difficulty concentrating. There is limited eye contact and body awareness may be greatly reduced. It is important to realize that this is not the persistent malaise associated with depression but that in this state, the client is truly "not present."

In a prolonged dorsal or sympathetic state, the ANS does not spring back to a ventral vagal state on its own. While we think of the sympathetic nervous system as the source of energetic charge, it can be confusing to consider that dorsal shutdown occurs *after* the sympathetic system has been activated but has not solved the problem. Frequently, as someone emerges from a state of dorsal shutdown, they feel a tremendous surge of energy as the body continues to process the survival energy produced in response to the threat.

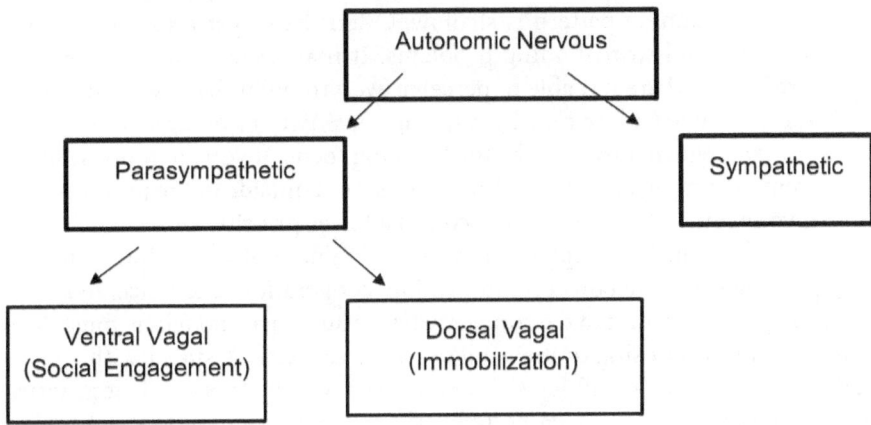

FIGURE 2.2
Elements of the Nervous System

Voice and Communication from a Polyvagal Perspective

The voice, both speaking and singing, plays an important role in the various states described above: in a ventral state, where there is social connection and security, the voice is relaxed, with a pleasant pitch (not too low or too high), melodious and prosodic. There is, partly due to the operation of the social engagement system, pleasant eye contact, relaxed breathing, and an alternation of listening and speaking among the interlocutors. In the singing voice, where there is interplay between the teacher, the singer, and other performers, there will be good coordination. In a sympathetic state, focused on survival through action and mobility, the mode is "fight/flight": the voice is characterized by increased overall muscle tension, speaking and singing is characterized by a quicker tempo, greater volume, often with more "staccato" or emphasis. The breathing pattern is high and accelerated. The client may unconsciously exert downward pressure on the tongue, or firmly press the tongue to the palate, and there is also often hypertonia (an abnormally high level of tension) of the masseter muscles, the diagonal muscles in the cheeks that contribute to chewing, both of which have consequences for mouth opening, vowel shapes, and sound formation. The singer in this state is less attuned to others. Their eyes will more often wander to their surroundings, continuing to scan for threats. Collaboration with other musicians may be more difficult, as the singer's system is primed to mobilize their building survival energy.

In a dorsal state, where immobility is the only available survival mode, there is withdrawal from contact. The muscle tone is "hypotonic" or slack; the voice becomes monotonous, flat, and often a little lower; speech is softer and slower. The breathing pattern is shallow. Often the singer also suffers from concentration and word-finding problems. It may seem as if they are "not quite present" and are not able to perceive everything in the environment. In both survival states, there may be a strong sensitivity to other sounds in the environment, which also disturbs the listening focus. If you are more attuned to movement among audience members or sound outside of the performance venue, your musical engagement becomes a lower priority.

In summary, the PVT explains how the body's natural survival states have a major biological impact on communication, cooperation, and voice. In a dorsal state, a singer cannot make contact with the audience and fellow musicians as easily and cannot sing to their full dynamic capacity. A singer with a sympathetic survival style will have difficulty with soft phonation, is less aware of themselves, and in some cases, may also provoke irritation in the listener.

Neuroception

The autonomic states described above are not caused by conscious reactions, but by unconscious perception of the environment, the inner state of the singer or speaker, and the corresponding unconscious reaction to it. Porges uses the word "neuroception" to describe the ways our neural pathways determine whether we are safe in a given situation.[17] Frequent Porges collaborator Stanley Rosenberg offers another definition:

> the unconscious processing by the ANS of information from the environment and the state of the body itself, is signaled by our senses. On the basis of this unconscious information, circuits in our body are activated: socially engaged in a safe and friendly environment (ventral vagal), defensive behavior when we feel threatened (sympathetic activation), and shutdown/conscious reduction when there is serious danger (dorsal vagal).[18]

Past experiences play a major role in these responses: a person who was lovingly raised and cared for by their parents as a child will default to a "neuroception of safety" through the experience of having friendly people who were helpful and involved. A person who was raised in a tense living environment, where there was a lot of arguing, shouting, and unpredictable parental behavior, is more likely to default to a neuroception of danger: the nervous system has learned to recognize these situations and constantly anticipates danger. As a result, these individuals are not likely to face the world confidently and are more likely to react with a sympathetic or dorsal response. The important takeaway for the singing teacher is that if your student is unable to engage with you socially before their lesson starts, signaling their status in a survival state, when we add in the stimulus of singing, they may quickly move into a state of freeze or dissociation, especially in the instance of traumatic coupling. As we'll see in chapter 7, it is interesting to note that in some cases, people can down-regulate or return to a ventral state by singing: feeling the voice vibrate in the body and prolonging their exhale. Considering Porges's hierarchy, establishing social engagement in the beginning of a lesson may help prepare students to tolerate the natural sympathetic activation that comes with the vulnerability of singing in front of others. If your student enters the studio in a state of heightened sympathetic activation, they may move into a dorsal response when the nervous system becomes even more stimulated. The singer's physical condition also plays a role: pain, chronic intestinal complaints, or hypersensitivity to sound can cause someone to have a continuously high level of nervous system activation and a feeling of insecurity.

In my practice I see people who have lived in threatening situations for a long time and have a default neuroception of danger. Based on their lived experiences and survival mode, they have learned to close themselves off from observing the physical world in real time. They "feel" less, because what they feel is too much for their system to process, and they have unconsciously learned to close themselves off from it. The same can be true for suppressing emotions. As we'll discuss in more depth in chapter 3, when emotions are not wanted or welcomed in the environment where someone grows up, suppressing them is an appropriate survival style. This also has a profound impact on the voice and on a singer's ability to engage in various emotional states as dictated by the music.

Co-Regulation

The last important aspect of the polyvagal theory is co-regulation.[19] Co-regulation is a psychological term that encapsulates the ways that humans are influenced by the nervous system states of others. A baby is safely "regulated" by their parents at a very young age: a parent hears from the way a baby cries whether it is hungry or has a dirty diaper and will respond appropriately depending on what the baby needs. This will reassure the baby and bring them into a ventral state. Children who are not comforted and are left alone for a long time are, in contrast, not regulated well and will eventually stop attempting to voice their needs (a dorsal response). Chapter 3 will dive into these conditions more deeply, but in the context of the polyvagal theory, let's look at two examples of the influence of nervous system states on others.

- A person who is agitated after an unpleasant conversation at work can come home angry (sympathetic) and calm down by taking his cat on his lap and stroking it. In this way the cat regulates his owner.
- Children in a class with a teacher who speaks quickly and loudly will unconsciously respond to this sympathetic activation. Depending on the imprint of the ANS of the individual children, in the face of this heightened energy they will either withdraw and not respond (dorsal response) or become very busy (sympathetic response).

Knowledge of co-regulation is essential for people who work with other people (and animals). This means that your state is influenced by the state of others: physically, emotionally, and even cognitively, the reverse is also true: your nervous system state can regulate others. A voice can activate and regulate. In this respect you can also think of the impact of a singer's voice on a listener. As teachers, you may be familiar with the sensation of sitting in the audience as one of your students performs. You are likely to be influenced by your student's state, and you may even feel more nervous than when you perform yourself. Take note that this exchange is reciprocal: if you approach your teaching with dread, frustration, or anger, no matter what you say or do to mask these feelings, your state will be perceptible to your student's nervous system. We'll discuss this further at the end of this chapter.

The Impact of Trauma

You'll recall from the introduction that the impact of trauma on body and mind has been described in the literature since the early twentieth century. Therapists who were confronted with soldiers who were severely traumatized in World War I saw people who could no longer move or speak. They described this phenomenon as "shell shock," but from the perspective of the polyvagal theory, we would now call this a dorsal reaction. German spiritual teacher Eckhart Tolle speaks of the link between body and mind, "the body is a representation of the unconscious mind. As a result, the trauma stored in your unconscious mind has a representation in the body." In my practice, I see daily that trauma experiences play a role in the background of misunderstood voice and throat problems.

A Case Study

Mieke is a sixty-two-year-old woman. Several years ago, she resigned from her work as a notary due to multiple physical complaints. She is not married and has no children. Five years ago, she suffered a serious heart attack, followed by breast cancer. Her voice has been bothering her for some time now; singing in a choir, which she loves, has become more and more difficult. The ENT diagnosed a "functional voice disorder": her vocal cords seem to work well. In our initial meeting, as she recounts her medical history, it appears that she is strongly focused on others: she is involved in the care of an aunt and that of her very elderly parents. This takes a lot of energy, but she also feels it is her duty. She is often congested and has chronic neck and shoulder pain. She has regular physical therapy for this and talks with a psychologist.

Her complaint consists of a sudden loss of voice; she says it feels as if there is a blockage in her throat, which makes it temporarily impossible for her to swallow and breathe. On palpation of the larynx, I feel tight, contracted laryngeal muscles. The larynx is strongly elevated. A massage of the laryngeal muscles gives her temporary relief. She seems to alternate between aphonia (loss of her ability to speak, which is a dorsal response), and a pinched voice (which indicates sympathetic arousal).

I express my suspicion that tensions play a role in the background. I explain to her how the nervous system works and also how her reactions to stressful situations can be explained. She confirms that her tensions have a lot to do with her parents. Her mother is a demanding woman; Mieke can't do anything right. This has been the case since her childhood: even when she got high marks for her studies, her mother was hardly satisfied. As a result, Mieke has also become demanding of herself. She is now permanently on call for her parents: her mother can call her three to four times a day to tell Mieke that something is wrong. Her father withdraws more and more and hardly reacts anymore to his wife. Mieke (still) doesn't dare go against her mother and goes to see her parents again and again to calm things down. When her father dies, her voice problems only increase, despite the fact that she is receiving ongoing treatment. She experiences more and more periods of aphonia which, understandably, is enormously difficult. I have contact with the psychologist who also doesn't know what to do. She has to go to the emergency room regularly for complaints of pain in her chest.

Then her mother also died suddenly. A month later I received a beautiful letter from her, in which she thanked me for my help and wrote that her voice had returned spontaneously after the death of her mother. She already sings with great pleasure in the choir again.

Applications of the Polyvagal Theory in Practice

I see many clients with unexplained complaints in the throat area, including many singers. My interest is the larynx and its connection with the social engagement system. The body is the basis of the voice, and the autonomic nervous system plays a major role in this, both in speaking and singing. In singers there can be greater sympathetic activation due to performance pressure and emotions, not only the singer's feelings about performing, self-doubt, and vulnerability, but also those related to the content of the music being sung.

In my experience in practice, clients feel understood by an explanation of the working of the nervous system and the polyvagal theory. They see that emotional, physical, and cognitive complaints are not "wrong," but the result of a dysregulation of their ANS. They recognize that this dysregulation has arisen around life events and difficulties or trauma. They become acquainted with the concepts of neuroplasticity and basic safety and experience that they can regulate themselves again after disruption. They see that "triggers" can elevate their symptoms and that by using internal and external resources, symptoms can diminish or even disappear completely.

Clients report that talking a lot about what they experienced can increase their complaints, but a body-oriented, nonjudgmental approach brings them further in terms of increasing nervous system capacity. At first, regulation may only be possible in the presence of a person with a quiet nervous system (co-regulation), but with time and continued exposure to safety, clients can learn to self-regulate in a healthy manner.

The Impact of Dysregulation on Voice and Other Complaints

Let's go back to the control of the various organ systems by the vagus nerve and the other cranial nerves involved in the ventral vagal complex.[20] As described above, the ventral vagus, along with four other cranial nerves, controls the eyes, jaw, facial muscles, throat, larynx, ears, heart, and lungs: the social engagement system. These muscles and organs are *supra-diaphragmatic,* or above the diaphragm.[21] The dorsal vagus controls the organs that are *sub-diaphragmatic*[22] or below the diaphragm: the digestive system and the sexual organs, for example. Rosenberg[23] writes in his book that in the field of anatomy it is usually not mentioned that the twelve cranial nerves have one thing in common: they are all related to finding food, chewing, swallowing, and digesting it, and eliminating undigested food. This means that a properly functioning autonomic system is responsible for communication *and* digestion. A dysregulated system therefore results in problems related to one or both systems.

In practice I see that many clients not only have voice problems but also intestinal problems such as irritable bowel syndrome (IBS). This insight has led me to adjust my assessment procedure, and I now ask for vision, voice, throat, hearing, heart, breathing, and digestive complaints as different symptoms of one system. A combination of a high, tense, loud speaking voice; hypertonic (rigid) laryngeal muscles; swallowing complaints; globus; rapid high breath and rapid heartbeat; and irritable bowel complaints points in the direction of chronic sympathetic activation. A combination of a low, soft/aphonic and monotone voice, with hypotonic (slack) laryngeal musculature, slow heart rate, shallow breath, and slow bowel function points toward a dorsal vagal condition. In addition, there is also a group of people who have symptoms of both patterns and vacillate between sympathetic and dorsal responses.

Porges developed the Body Perception Questionnaire (BPQ[24]), a questionnaire that measures the occurrence of physical symptoms and classifies them into supra- and subdiaphragmatic symptoms. I administered this questionnaire in a study to fifty-four new clients[25] in the practice and compared their scores with the scores of people in a control group. Analysis showed that people with voice and throat complaints had significantly more supradiaphragmatic symptoms than people in the control group. This may explain why people with voice complaints also have other complaints of muscle groups and functions of the ventral vagal complex. Much research is still needed into questions that arise from these insights.

Voice and Trauma

Porges did not initially focus on the field of trauma therapy when designing and describing his theory. Since the appearance of Porges's first publication on PVT,[26] however, his theory has been embraced by several founders of body-oriented trauma therapy. Peter Levine, the creator of the body-oriented therapy *somatic experiencing* describes trauma as "an unfinished movement,"[27] a movement that is blocked in the body and can still be discharged. Bessel van der Kolk, a psychiatrist working in the United States, uses fMRI scans to investigate how connections in the brain are disrupted by trauma and what the effects are on cognition, emotion, and behavior.[28] The pictures of these scans speak volumes, very clearly showing the differences in brain activity in sympathetic and dorsal vagal states. The current view from the perspective of body-oriented trauma therapy is that the effects of trauma are stored in the nervous system in the form of dysregulation,[29] making the ventral vagal state temporarily unavailable.

Because the basis for many traumas was laid in early childhood, in a period in which language was not yet fully developed, talking about what happened often does not have the desired effect. After all, language was not sufficiently developed at the time. If the consequence of trauma creates a chronic dorsal state, there is also little language available. The good news is that we now know that brains are neuroplastic and that recovery is possible through the construction of new connections in the brain.

Body-Oriented Approach

A body-centered approach helps the client become aware of physical reactions to triggers. However, many people have little body awareness. An example of this is that a person may dissociate in a threatening situation and therefore not feel their body, which can be a perfectly appropriate response to the moment and also lifesaving. However, this dorsal pattern of dissociating during a tense situation, can still be active years after the initial event and is then no longer functional. When, during body-oriented therapy, clients consciously experience their jaw tension, tight throat, and restricted breath, this can sometimes lead to spontaneous discharges, resulting in involuntary movements of their bodies. This connects to the "unfinished movement" as Levine describes it:[30] the movement that was impossible at the time can still be carried out by the body after the fact. In this way, emotions held back for years can still be released.

For the singing teacher or speech therapist, the priority is to offer safety and support. Continuing to ask questions of a client and requiring them to talk about their trauma carries the danger of re-traumatization, is counterproductive, and also unnecessary. After releasing stored tensions in the body, the voice can often spontaneously sound free and open again.

Re-Regulating the Autonomic Nervous System

A healthy ANS is able to re-regulate itself after phases of heightened sympathetic activation. People who have gone through a severe experience and have persistent symptoms are often no longer able to regulate themselves. They are in a prolonged state of survival: either activated, with a high level of arousal, or in a state of shutdown, immobilized.

There are several inputs by which the ANS can be regulated:

1. The Autonomic State of the Practitioner

You are the instrument by which the singer can be "re-regulated." To radiate safety by means of your own ventral state, expressed by your facial expression, voice, breathing, muscle tension, and mood is a prerequisite for this. Clients are extremely sensitive to signals that indicate danger: the neuroception of clients is sharply tuned based on the imprint of their ANS, thus they also react to the state of the therapist. A nonjudgmental reflective attitude is the starting point.

It is necessary to be able to regulate your own state as a therapist/coach, even if the client may be telling an intense story. Therapists and teachers must therefore recognize and be able to regulate their own physical, emotional, and cognitive patterns.

2. Psychoeducation

Explaining the functioning of the ANS and its different states can help the client recognize which autonomic state they are in. Social worker and polyvagal educator Deb Dana is the author of numerous resources to help practitioners apply the principles of the polyvagal theory in their practice, including *Polyvagal Exercises for Safety and Connection*, *The Polyvagal Flip Chart*, *Anchored*, and courses on her website (https://rhythmofregulation.com). Dana has developed and published several tools that can be used to help people recognize the characteristics of their different autonomous states.

When the client can look at this without judgment, the practitioner can work with the client to find the triggers that activate their state. Then the client can learn to recognize resources that will help them to calm down and regulate.

3. Exercises to Regulate the Nervous System

- Prolonged exhalation
- Singing, as this also results in a long expiration
- Grounding and breathing exercises, such as yoga, qigong
- Moving, walking, playing sports, dancing, singing, in order to drain and discharge accumulated nervous system energy
- Spending time in nature
- Listening to soothing or activating music, depending on the state and musical preference of the client
- Safe and Sound Protocol (SSP)

The Safe and Sound Protocol (SSP) is an auditory therapy developed by Porges aimed at calming the ANS.[31] Porges explains that the state of our autonomic nervous system is strongly determined by sound. To understand this, first, here is a brief explanation of how hearing works:

Sound is captured by the eardrum and transmitted through a chain of ossicles and muscles located in the middle ear to the inner ear, where it is interpreted. The muscle tension in the middle ear regulates the tension of the eardrum, and depending on its tension, like a drum, specific sounds can be picked up.

To be in a ventral state, it is important to be able to understand people in the vicinity well. Sounds that fit in with this, such as the melody and prosody of a relaxed human voice, must then be able to be transmitted and interpreted by the inner ear and autonomic nervous system accordingly. In a sympathetic state, in which mammals must be able to respond quickly to external signals of danger, the auditory system is keen on specific sounds. Porges describes[32] that in this state these are particularly the higher and shrill sounds. In a dorsal state there is a different sensitivity to sound: here it is mainly low and booming sounds that can indicate danger of life and generate the corresponding autonomic reaction. In a sympathetic or dorsal state, there is therefore a different muscle tension in the middle ear than in a ventral state because people are more focused on sounds in the environment. When people are exposed to life-threatening danger for a long time, their autonomic state can persist for a long time. This also has consequences for hearing.

Prolonged exposure to danger can cause people to have more difficulty following a relaxed conversation, and to be very sensitive to environmental sounds. Auditory hypersensitivity is often the result of this. I see many people with a dysregulated autonomic nervous system who are very sensitive to sound in their environment and therefore cannot function well. This can also be troublesome for singers who have to work together with varying voices or instruments.

Porges has developed the Safe and Sound Protocol[33] to calm the autonomic nervous system by listening to vocal music from which "sympathetic and dorsal" sound has been filtered out. Clients listen to SSP under the supervision of a trained therapist for one hour at a time, several days in a row. During listening, stuck physical and emotional patterns can become conscious and move again.

At the request of Dr. Porges, I researched the effect of the application of this program in people with functional voice and throat complaints.[34] It appeared that after treatment with SSP, voice and throat complaints decreased significantly, and autonomic dysregulation and anxiety decreased significantly. The analysis of the participants' voices prior to and after the intervention is still ongoing. The observation from clients is that many complaints such as chronic jaw tension seem to disappear spontaneously.

A Case Study to Illustrate the Effect of SSP

Marc is a singer, forty-eight years old. He has been a professional lead singer in a big band for quite some time and is having increasing difficulty singing loud and high. He also suffers from tinnitus, which often prevents him from hearing the music well. He tells us that he also had a breakdown before a recent performance and was very shocked by it. It also made him anxious. The band has regular tours, which cause him so much trouble that he is considering quitting singing. On examination, I notice that there is tremendous hypertonia in the laryngeal region and in his neck. More symptoms of autonomic dysregulation also emerge: he suffers from IBS, sleeps poorly, and is often restless.

In consultation, we decided to try SSP. We made five appointments for the following week to listen to the music for an hour every day under remote guidance. He visibly enjoys this and reports that he experiences a deep relaxation while listening. He becomes aware of his restlessness and the tension in his neck and chest and can let go of it more and more. His tension decreases in the course of the week. He also gets more enjoyment out of voice exercises again. He discovers that he can maintain calm by taking long walks.

Shortly after the SSP, another tour starts. While adjusting the sound system, the sound engineer notices that the setting of Marc's earphones needs to be completely changed. As a result, he can hear the music much better and also notices that the disturbing tinnitus has disappeared.

The Role of the Clinician

In situations where there is trauma in the background, body-oriented trauma therapy is desirable. Each of us must always bear in mind our own ethical scope of practice. A singing teacher can have concerns about vocal health based on their expertise but must refer to an ENT for a diagnosis. Remember that ENTs and speech pathologists refer to mental health professionals when they suspect a psychogenic voice disorder. If you are not also trained in trauma healing therapy, it is not ethical or responsible for you to attempt to engage with a singer's trauma, though you are encouraged to consider using the principles of nervous system regulation to create an environment of safety for all singers. Chapter 4 includes brief descriptions of several known healing modalities. People can start to experience that survival patterns were functional in the past but are no longer required in the present. After that, a ventral state with corresponding voice possibilities can become available again. Encouraging people to speak out and develop new speaking habits is often not necessary at all. In a ventral state, when someone feels safe, these behaviors arise naturally. When clients get to know their own nervous system, and can regulate and calm themselves, complaints seem to disappear spontaneously. When someone has been functioning in a sympathetic state for years and learns to communicate ventrally, the breathing pattern can spontaneously change, the diaphragm can function optimally again, and the larynx and jaw can relax. This results in a reduction of complaints. If necessary, vocal exercises can then be given to more quickly achieve an optimal effect. The question arises whether and how this can be addressed in the treatment of clients with functional voice complaints.

Speech therapists, singing teachers and other professionals will recognize that tension and stress play a role in the background of voice complaints. However, they are not trained to treat these aspects, which play a central role in the dysregulation of the autonomic nervous system and the development of voice disorders. ENTs will refer clients with psychogenic voice disorders to psychologists. The problem with this is that many psychologists don't have knowledge of voice problems. Because of the prevalence of trauma, we advocate that speech therapists and other voice professionals be trained in trauma informed practice. It is not the practitioner's responsibility to heal the singer's trauma; it is our role to regulate our own systems so they convey safety, to offer support to singers if they disclose that they have experienced trauma, and to know some of the most common signs of trauma so that we can recognize and help to rebalance their ANS when a nervous system may be in distress.

Notes

1. S. Porges, "Orienting in a Defensive World: Mammalian Modifications of Our Evolutionary Heritage: A Polyvagal Theory," *International Journal of Psychophysiology* 32, no. 4 (1995): 301–18.

2. S. W. Porges, *Polyvagal Safety, Attachment, Communication, Self-Regulation* (W.W. Norton & Company, 2021), introduction, page xx.

3. J. Baker, *Psychosocial Perspectives in the Management of Voice Disorders* (Compton Publishing Ltd., 2017), 6–11.

4. Ibid.

5. Ibid.

6. L. W. Baijens, R. Verdonschot, S. Vanbelle, et al., "Medically Unexplained Otorhinolaryngological Symptoms: Towards Integrated Psychiatric Care," *Laryngoscope* 125 (2015):1583–87.

7. B. Hellinger, *Familien stellen mit Kranken* (Carl Auer Verlag, 1998).

8. G. Weber and S. Hausner, *Praxis der Systemaufstellung* (2009), 65–73.

9. Somatic Experiencing International, https://traumahealing.org.

10. S. W. Porges, *The Polyvagal Theory: Neurophysiological Foundations of Emotions, Attachment, Communication and Self Regulation* (W.W. Norton & Company, 2011).

11. Ibid.

12. S. W. Porges, *Polyvagal Safety, Attachment, Communication, Self-Regulation* (W.W. Norton & Company, 2021), 1–11.
13. Porges, "Orienting in a Defensive World," 301–18.
14. Porges, *Polyvagal safety, attachment, communication, self-regulation*, 208–10.
15. Ibid., 208–30.
16. Ibid.
17. Ibid., 11–19.
18. S. Rosenberg, *Accessing the Healing Power of the Vagus Nerve* (North Atlantic Books, 2017), p. 41 [Dutch translation].
19. D. Dana, *The Polyvagal Theory in Therapy* (W.W. Norton & Company, 2018), 44–47.
20. Porges, *Polyvagal Safety, Attachment, Communication, Self-regulation*, 32.
21. Ibid.
22. Ibid., 19.
23. Rosenberg, *Accessing the Healing Power of the Vagus Nerve*, 1–27.
24. J. Kolacz, G. F. Lewis, O. Roath, et al. (preliminary citation, article in preparation), "The Body Perception Questionnaire Short Form: Norms and Association with Objective Lab Assessments," 2020. The BPQ can be found on the website of Dr. Porges: https://www.stephenporges.com
25. Article under review.
26. Porges, "Orienting in a Defensive World," 301–18.
27. P. A. Levine, *Waking the Tiger, Healing Trauma* (North Atlantic Books, 2008).
28. B. van der Kolk, *The Body Keeps the Score: Brain, Mind and Body in Healing of Trauma* (Penguin, 2014).
29. Van der Kolk, *The Body Keeps the Score*.
30. Levine, *Waking the Tiger, Healing Trauma*.
31. Porges, *The Polyvagal Theory*, 202–14.
32. Ibid.
33. Ibid.
34. Article under review.

3

Attachment and Developmental Trauma

Emily Jaworski Koriath

Human beings are a social species; the need to connect to others is part of our biological wiring, and the human attachment system is where that wiring resides.[1] Attachment theory seeks to codify patterns of human behavior and how they are affected by our original relationship blueprint, that of infant and caregiver.[2]

British psychologist John Bowlby, the first to introduce the theory of attachment in the 1940s, was influenced by his own personal history of being raised by a nanny and then sent away to boarding school at the age of seven. After he completed his studies, Bowlby began working at the Child Guidance Clinic of London, where he studied the distress of children separated from their mothers. Some of the boys in the center were placed there because of criminal behavior, and Bowlby designed studies to determine how the boys' developmental history could potentially be linked to their behavior issues.[3] In 1950, Bowlby was joined by psychologist Mary Ainsworth, who served as a research assistant to Bowlby before branching out to conduct her own research. By 1965, Ainsworth had developed what she called the Strange Situation Procedure, which was designed as the first instrument to gather empirical data to support Bowlby's theories.[4]

For this study, Ainsworth had mothers and their children (aged twelve to twenty-four months) enter a pleasant room with toys and other distractions for the child. After a set period, a stranger would enter the room, interact with the mother, and attempt to interact with the child. At another specified interval, the mother would leave the room, leaving the child with the stranger.

Ainsworth found that some of the children became instantly distressed at the mother's absence but were easily soothed upon her return. Some children became distressed but could not be soothed, even when the mother returned. Still another group showed no reaction upon the mother's exit or reentry. Based on the results of these studies, Ainsworth began to group children into three categories: *secure, anxious,* and *avoidant*.[5, 6, 7] One of Ainsworth's students, Mary Main, published a fourth attachment style, *disorganized attachment*, in 1986.[8]

Under ideal circumstances, we would grow up with what is known as *secure attachment*. People who demonstrate secure attachment grew up with plenty of love and support from consistently responsive caregivers. As adults, they are interdependent, connecting with others in healthy, mutually beneficial ways. According to a 1986 paper by Mary Main, "children judged secure . . . have repeatedly been found to be more cooperative, more empathic, and more competent than children who were judged insecure."[9] But when our care is inconsistent, ineffective, or downright dangerous, we develop one of three attachment adaptations.[10] In *The Power of Attachment,* therapist Diane Poole Heller explains that if we are not raised in an environment where secure attachment is available to us, we have more difficulty developing trust for others, and it's harder to ask for help or even *think* of asking for help.[11] As an infant, if you cried to let someone know that you needed help and no help was offered to you, you might assume that help will *never* be available. As psychologist Maureen Gallagher explains, "attachment adaptations are survival adaptations," because human infants cannot survive without external sources of care. Our developing brains adapt quickly to the care that is available to us in order to ensure our survival.

Attachment and Communication

In 2021, Anna Rupert and Diane Bartlett published the results of an extensive survey of speech pathologists' knowledge of the link between childhood trauma and attachment and communication development. At the time of the survey, numerous studies had been published (dating as far back as 1982) that demonstrate that trauma exposure affects communication development in children. Those who had experienced maltreatment had "significantly poorer speech and language abilities in terms of receptive, expressive, and pragmatic language skills when compared to children who had not experienced maltreatment."[12] As we read in chapter 1, trauma exposure has also been shown to negatively impact problem solving, memory, executive functioning, sensory modulation, emotional regulation, and intellectual functioning, which are all important to communication development.

For children, communication skills are learned in the context of back-and-forth interactions with a caregiver, a process known as "serve and return"; a child attempts to make contact with a caregiver, "serving" a babble, a coo, or eye contact. The caregiver "returns the serve" as in a game of tennis, by talking back, playing peek-a-boo, or otherwise engaging with the child.[13] But when trauma occurs within the child-caregiver relationship, this process is disrupted, inconsistent, or not present, which can directly impact language acquisition.

The survey instrument used in the study revealed that deeper awareness of childhood trauma and attachment needs to be universally integrated and understood across the field of speech pathology. Rupert advocates that SLP practitioners should develop a comprehensive understanding of trauma and attachment, symptomology, and impacts, because without it, they may "miss many opportunities for prevention, identification, and providing trauma-informed care." On the other hand, "SLP practitioners who fully understand attachment and the benefits beyond language learning will be better equipped to provide coaching that improves the attachment relationship and, therefore, produces impacts beyond improving communication skills."

This perspective is beginning to take hold internationally, as both the Royal College of Speech and Language Therapists in the United Kingdom, and SLP Australia have recently expanded training guidelines to include knowledge of attachment and trauma, family systems, and trauma theory. As of this writing, neither organization has yet provided specific guidelines for the ways that practice should be altered.

The study results and subsequent recommendations are echoed by Howard Steele, professor of psychology and founding president of the Society for Emotion and Attachment Studies, who says that when it comes to monitoring a person's speech patterns, a clinician's responsibility

> is to focus both on what is said, and how "it" is said, especially when "it" refers to loss or trauma. Lapses in the monitoring of speech (being inconsistent re: time or space) or reason (describing a dead person in the present tense OR claiming an abuser acted out of concern to teach valuable lessons), and excessive attention to detail (absorption) are linked to unresolved loss or unresolved trauma, with follow-on effects of frightened or frightening caregiving behavior that is typically highly dysregulating to infants.[14]

The perspectives emerging from both speech pathology and the psychology of attachment suggest that those of us who work in the field of expressive communication (including singing) can better serve our clients (students) by understanding that there are numerous factors that can impact a person's ability to communicate effectively and clearly. It's not hard to imagine that if everyday speech is affected by attachment trauma, the heightened communication and intense vulnerability required for artistic presentation may be challenging to acquire for many students. As Rupert suggests, the role of the clinician is to offer a strong opportunity for attachment in the context of their prescribed work with a student, thereby offering an opportunity for safe exploration of the possibilities of expression.

You may also be sensing the relevance that attachment has to our deeply personal, one-on-one work with singers and clients in the studio or clinic. The manner a person has adapted to interact with others will no doubt be replicated in our relationship to them. The good news is that, just like trauma, we never need to know the origins of a singer's adaptations, and the descriptions provided below are not an invitation to guess someone else's attachment style or make assumptions about their needs. Secure adaptation is biologically imprinted in us, and thanks to the wonders of neuroplasticity, we can recall it and excavate it.[15] This means that in the voice studio, therapy room, or clinic, the work that you do to create healthy attachment with your clients can be transformative and healing and transfer to their other relationships. By practicing secure attachment skills, we can provide an opportunity for our clients to learn co-regulation in the presence of a healthy adult and move toward what's known as "earned secure."

Studies show that for secure attachment to develop, babies need to be in emotional attunement with their caregivers only 30 percent of the time. As Poole Heller says, "Nobody needs to be perfect for deep and lasting healing" to occur.[16] Let's investigate the three types of attachment adaptations and how they may make themselves known in your relationships with singers. Information on building secure attachment skills can be found in part 2.

Exercise 3.1

Journal prompts can help you gain insight into your attachment style.

Below are a few questions inspired by the *Adult Attachment Interview*, a series of questions first published in 1985 by George, Kaplan, and Main at the University of California, Berkeley, and by the Adverse Childhood Experiences questionnaire developed by the Centers for Disease Control. Both tools are available online in their entirety.[17,18] This is not a diagnostic psychological tool and is only meant to give you direction in exploring your past and thinking about how adaptation exists for you currently.

1. *Family structure and circumstances*
   What do you know about your family's* history? Where were you born? Where were your parents born? Who were your caregivers? Did your

family unit live together or in a few different places? Were there important people in your life who lived far away? Did you move around a lot? Did adults in your life work outside the home?
2. *Household challenges*
Did you ever witness violence in your home? Did anyone in your family misuse substances of any kind? Did anyone that you grew up with have a mental illness that you know of? Did you lose any important people in your life while you were growing up? They may have been significant to you personally, like a friend or close relative, or you may not have known them well, but they were significant to a caregiver.
3. *Climate of care*
When you were upset as a child, what did you do? What about if you were hurt physically? To which of your caregivers were you closest, and why? What adjectives would you use to describe the environment in which you grew up?
4. Looking back on your answers, can you see any themes emerging, or memories that you'd forgotten? How do you think that your upbringing relates to the way you interact with others in your adult life?

*For the sake of brevity, in the above questions, "family" is used for the group of people among whom you were raised, including but not limited to adult caregivers of any number or gender, and any other children present in your home most of the time.

Avoidant Attachment

What Is It?

Folks with avoidant attachment may be viewed as always keeping their distance from others. They may also project an attitude that relationships are not important or even necessary. The most common contributors to the development of an avoidant adaptation are isolation, absence of touch, emotional neglect, or what Poole Heller refers to as "task-based presence"; the caregiver is present, but only when the infant is practical or functional. You can imagine this behavior manifesting in adolescence in parents who only recognize their children when they are achieving something.[19]

How Might It Show Up in Singers?

For most people who have developed an avoidant attachment style, their predominant experience in childhood was unresponsiveness. They cried but were not soothed, or they were left alone for too long. Because of this, you may see your students working to appear stoic at all costs. If you ask them what questions they have, they may respond with silence. They will likely not engage with any pre-lesson conversation, as they are most concerned with following the standard procedure, or accomplishing things based on goals they've set. This independence and sometimes extreme self-reliance are not exclusively negative; we must remember that students come to us based on the way their brains developed in response to their care. Their behaviors worked to keep them alive, and they have managed to appear before you trying to sing. It may be difficult for these singers to tap into a larger sense of purpose, or why they have committed to singing; when I ask seemingly disinterested singers why they have chosen to study music, some students tell me that they're "not good at anything else," and so may not identify with attempts to tap into passion or deep feeling. In early stages of study, emotional connection will be difficult. They will be most focused on learning music accurately and may show little physical response to the music. These students will not likely respond to abstract descriptions of concepts or metaphors as a teaching tool.

You may describe these folks as detached, off in their own world, insensitive, cold, or standoffish.[20] Those with the avoidant adaptation learn to stop reaching out for help because they don't expect others to be there or meet their needs.[21] For teachers, it can be useful to offer even the simplest of reframes; instead of asking "Do you have any questions?" try asking "What questions do you have?" This subtle shift in language hints that questions would be normal and expected at any given stage in the work. Over time, such habits in a teacher begin to establish a sense of safety and continuity for the student. They learn that they don't need to be perfect to gain approval, and that the teacher's presence is not conditional. Reconnecting to others in safe and healthy ways is extremely important for people who have developed an avoidant attachment style.

This is where the teacher's wellness becomes crucial; what would it take for you to commit to each student for as long as they study with you? It may be helpful to consider clear, frequently communicated policies like announcing your absences well in advance, or scheduling conversations if a change in studio placement becomes necessary. Keep semester goals and lesson objectives clear so students know when they are meeting expectations. You are not being asked to lower your standards or to "baby" your students. Communicating boundaries and expectations clearly and effectively benefits everyone.

With the release of her third book, *The Singer's Epiphany*, it became public knowledge that my doctoral mentor Dr. Lynn Eustis has faced significant health challenges in recent years, including surgery for a massive abdominal tumor, which happened to occur during my doctoral studies. At the beginning of the semester, in which she would be on leave to have surgery and recover, she emailed each of her students and communicated a detailed plan about missed lessons, and sessions with professional staff accompanists to make sure that we all continued learning and would be well prepared for our required performances. She managed this absence so well that *I forgot that it happened* until I read about it in her book. This is the goal: you are a human with all of your very human needs and wants, and you also consider how your actions will affect others. You are not responsible for excavating or healing their childhood wounds, but your presence and communication can go a long way in establishing and maintaining a sense of trust and relationship continuity.

In lessons, and perhaps most especially onstage when the body goes into survival energy, be aware that dissociation could be a likely response to intense nervous system activation for the student with avoidant attachment. Checking out or viewing yourself from a distance is a deactivating strategy, upon which some avoidant folks may rely when stress is high.[22] It's too hard to need something from another and not get it, so sometimes people dissociate so they can't feel how much this hurts. In *Trauma and Dissociation in a Cross-Cultural Perspective,* Vedat Sar and Erdinc Ozturk offer a clear and helpful definition of dissociation: traumatic experiences and the altered self-perception that results make it harder for our internal world to match external reality.[23] Students may lose the ability to hear auditory cues clearly, or to count accurately, or to tune to the piano. I was conducting a musical and needed to have a conversation with an actor who consistently missed a musical cue. As we tried to analyze the situation, he hypothesized that this particular cue was especially difficult because the other actors onstage were screaming during the scene. I acknowledged that such distractions do indeed present obstacles, and I assured him that we could make eye contact, and I would give him a point and a reassuring nod when it was time for him to sing. However, when we next ran the scene, I noticed that in truth, there was no other noise onstage during this scene. The actor's internal perception did not match reality.

Some people with avoidant attachment may manifest deep discomfort with eye contact,[24] because it signals need or suggests emotional intimacy. It's best for practitioners to be gentle with demanding eye contact, and to allow singers to move in and out of it as they feel comfortable. In this way, you give the student permission to honor their own instincts and needs, without demanding something that could force them into a vulnerable position. Even this level of choice can signal acceptance and subtly influence the nervous system.[25] An easy cue is "you can let your eyes go wherever they want."

Avoidant folks are often used to being alone and can become deeply involved in their own personal experience. It takes time to adjust out of this, and transitions can be difficult. For this reason, it's helpful to have a chat with your students about their schedule. Do they come to you after a quiet morning or an afternoon nap? If they are rushing to work with you after a heavy morning of academic coursework, they may need some social engagement to be able to relate to you honestly and drop into their work. An especially useful tactic are questions about the observable world: How is the weather? How was your walk to the building? What did you see? By helping the singer orient themselves to their physical surroundings, the practitioner can gently call them out of their internal depths.

Anxious Attachment

What Is It?

People with anxious attachment (also called *ambivalent attachment* in some sources) are not secure in the belief that they are loved, and may not even believe that they are lovable, because their care was either intermittent or wholly unpredictable. These students will demonstrate anxiety about having their needs met and may become convinced that being abandoned by others is inevitable. As an infant, if you don't know who will show up, or if your needs will be met, it creates anxiety, doubt, insecurity, and a lot of additional stress on top of the stress caused by your original need. The good news is that if a singer has a wound related to consistency, your stability, reliability, and reassurance as their teacher will go a long way toward easing their fear.

In essence, these singers are always looking for someone to come and help, to soothe, to fix. They may be seen as complainers, but this is a survival adaptation. Positive thinking or well-intentioned platitudes will not help this student and in fact may make them feel even more alone and misunderstood. This person is deeply afraid that they will lose the people who care for them. They may display numerous cries for attention, or a pressurized word flow (talking too much or too fast or with too many hard-to-follow details). Sometimes this "signal cry" manifests through the body in chronic illness or myriad ailments—the body gets involved in crying for help when other behaviors aren't enough.

How Does It Show Up in Singers?

Again, we learn about healthy emotional regulation from the models we have access to growing up. The first step to emotional self-regulation is experiencing regulation externally; if you grow up with secure attachment, your caregivers help you learn to navigate your changing emotions while they remain present and supportive. But if children don't experience consistent and reliable external regulation, they will not be able to develop an internal regulation system. Because of this, you might be tempted to describe a singer as needy, clingy, or high maintenance.[26] They may fret over what you might consider trivial details like where to park or the location of the restrooms. They may refuse to put down their water bottles, or they may sip almost compulsively as you work. They are constantly looking for others to calm or soothe them because they haven't figured out how to soothe themselves.[27]

It's important for us as teachers of the arts to know that people with ambivalent attachment have often developed incredible sensitivity to their environments. They read the people around them for indications of mood and read deeply into interactions with others. On the one hand, this type of sensitivity and empathy can serve performing artists well. But without an awareness of attachment adaptations, we may also view these same students as *overly sensitive* (meaning that they are easily wounded by what the teacher views as necessary, constructive feedback). By no means does this suggest that we cannot offer feedback to a particular subset of students, but if you suspect that a student has developed anxious attachment, your support and continued presence will be crucial in helping them to learn that critique does not mean abandonment. More information on feedback strategies appears in chapter 7.

Disorganized Attachment

What Is It?

Disorganized attachment wasn't part of Mary Ainsworth's original publications on attachment theory; her former doctoral student, psychologist Mary Main, first published on disorganized attachment in 1986 in a chapter of *Affective Development in Infancy*.[28] Main and her team carefully examined the video footage of the children from Ainsworth's original Strange Situation Procedure who were deemed "unclassifiable," many of whom were notably maltreated by their caregivers.

When a caregiver is the source of fear, or an infant is subjected to ongoing emotional turmoil, the attachment system becomes entangled with survival instincts. This can result in extreme hypervigilance, or a constant orientation toward threats; self-absorption, controlling behaviors, and a tendency to lash out.[29] The disorganized attachment style is difficult to track and presents with fewer obvious characteristics than the other attachment adaptations. Perhaps the best way to know if you're working with someone who has adapted a disorganized style is that you can't tuck them into any other category.[30] This singer is basically in chronic overarousal, which the body deals with in one of two ways: constant fight-or-flight, or total shut down. This can manifest as lack of motivation, disconnection or spacing out, poor impulse control, and under-performance in school.

As kids, they may act out their distress and get labeled as "problem children" and then they get punished by their teachers or other authority figures, and the cycle of misattunement continues. In the extreme, this can lead to addiction, psychiatric conditions, personality disorders, and criminal behaviors. You're less likely to encounter this student in a voice lesson setting unless they have already begun to heal from some of their early wounds. When I was working in a community music school, I was assigned a new student that we'll call Agnes. While initial student meetings can often be awkward, I could usually find a way to get some usable information to build a strategy upon. Not so with Agnes. She couldn't provide a single direct answer to any of my questions, including "What kind of music do you like?" and "What seems interesting about voice lessons?" After I finished teaching for the night, my supervisor pulled me aside to let me know that Agnes had been hospitalized several times for intense psychological treatment and self-harming behaviors but had just been placed with a new foster family and all signs looked positive. It was this foster family who had heard Agnes singing in her room; they encouraged her to take voice lessons as a way of cultivating her interest and building a positive home environment. It took me and Agnes several weeks to settle into a rapport, and through a lot of discussion and trial and error, we settled on two different pop songs to work on, which Agnes was already singing well. I thought we could keep building our momentum (and Agnes's sense of security and confidence) and eventually expand into new repertoire.

The following week, I looked forward to Agnes's lesson, feeling that we had turned a corner together and could begin to work in a new way. But Agnes arrived sullen and almost nonresponsive. She was picking at her jewelry in a repetitive way and wouldn't meet my eyes. After a lot of quiet, Agnes told me that she didn't like any of the songs we had chosen, and she didn't want to sing them. I thanked her for her honesty and scheduled another repertoire exploration for the following week. That's when Agnes let me know that she had found a new church that was incredibly meaningful to her, and she wanted to focus on music she could sing for her newfound community. After about three weeks of noticeable improvement in a variety of styles, Agnes came into her lesson saying that she didn't want to sing any of those songs anymore either. A week after that, she stopped coming to her lessons altogether.

Without knowing the full details of Agnes's history, I could still see that what was happening in our studio relationship had essentially nothing to do with me. Agnes was a teenager who was still trying to find a family. There were some dissociative behaviors on display (like her picking at her jewelry and "zoning out" while we talked), and while this was before my official trauma training began, I could see that my role in Agnes's life at that moment in time was to accept her in whatever state she entered the studio, listen to her ideas about music and using her voice, and sing with her when she was ready to sing.

If you are lucky enough to grow up with secure attachment, you learn healthy co-regulation and internal regulation (or "self-regulation"). You learn co-regulation first from the healthy models around you, and as you develop, you also develop the ability to self-regulate. You are loved and supported, and you can recover from being upset more quickly. As Diane Poole Heller describes it, you end up with "a lot of relational resilience because these two forms of regulation are appropriately developed, available, and in balance."[31]

Not so with the avoidant and anxious adaptations. Neither group received satisfying or consistent interactive regulation, but they adapted in different ways. Avoidant people couldn't count on others to help them and so they lose the sense of the other. You don't have a reliable imprint of what co-regulation looks like, so you stop looking to others for help, and develop a mindset that you are on your own. Anxiously attached people are primed to seek soothing from others to the exclusion of self-regulation. They want someone to take care of them, and they lose their sense of self. Avoidant folks find balance by learning to let others in and finding healthy forms of supportive connection; anxious folks can heal by developing a firmer sense of self and learning to self-soothe. Disorganized folks can't self-soothe *or* be soothed by others.[32]

How Might It Show Up in Singers?

A singer with disorganized attachment will probably not be interested in connecting to an audience, especially at first, since their earliest attempts at connecting to others were coupled with fear. It may also be difficult for these students to be free and responsive to the music; control has been an important part of survival. This person developed a mindset in infancy that said, "If I can control everything, then I can stay safe." Letting go can be terrifying since controlling elements of their environment has helped them to survive. Be ready to be patient with expressive skills and to work slowly on helping the student to build tolerance of the natural fight or flight energy that gets activated onstage. They may experience heightened nervous system states just by being with you in the studio. In these singers, that energy is over-coupled with survival response; these are the students who might start to feel as though they will die onstage because historically in their body, that level of nervous system activation came on in response to literal threats to their life. You may see reactions to performance energy that don't make obvious sense to you.

These students will probably also present with a lack of self-worth and a persistent feeling of being a failure. This is heartbreaking but makes sense considering their past. When they were growing up, nothing they did could protect them or prevent bad things from happening. Over time, it's only natural that such conditions would erode your confidence and your belief that you can create change.

Notes

1. Mary D. Salter Ainsworth, "Attachments beyond Infancy," *American Psychologist* 44 no. 4, 709.

2. Inge Bretherton, "The Origins of Attachment Theory: John Bowlby and Mary Ainsworth," *Developmental Psychology* 28, no. 5 (1992) 762–63

3. Ibid., 759–60.

4. Lenny Van Rosmalen, René Van Der Veer, and Frank Van Der Horst, "Ainsworth's Strange Situation Procedure: The Origin of an Instrument," *Journal of the History of the Behavioral Sciences* 51, no. 3 (2015).

5. Bretherton "The Origins of Attachment Theory," 765.

6. Van Rosmalen et al., "Ainsworth's Strange Situation Procedure," 278.

7. Mary D. Salter Ainsworth and Silvia M. Bell, "Attachment, Exploration, and Separation: Illustrated by the Behavior of One-Year-Olds in a Strange Situation," *Child Development* 41, no. 1 (1970): 49–67. https://doi.org/10.2307/1127388.

8. T. Berry Brazelton and Michael W. Yogman, eds., *Affective Development in Infancy* (Ablex Publishing Company, 1986).

9. Mary Main and Judith Solomon, "Discovery of an Insecure-Disorganized/Disoriented Attachment Pattern," in *Affective Development in Infancy*, edited by T. B. Brazelton and M. W. Yogman (Ablex Publishing Company, 1986).

10. Diane Poole Heller, *The Power of Attachment: How to Create Deep and Lasting Intimate Relationships* (Boulder: Sounds True, 2019), 57.

11. Ibid., 7.

12. Research by Allen and Oliver, 1982; Coster and Cicchetti, 1993; Coster et al., 1989; Culp et al., 1991; Law and Conway, 1992; Rogers-Adkinson and Stuart, 2007; Spratt et al., 2012; Stacks et al., 2011. Summarized in Anna C. Rupert and Diane E Bartlett, "The Childhood Trauma and Attachment Gap in Speech-Language Pathology: Practitioner's Knowledge, Practice, and Needs," *American Journal of Speech-Language Pathology* 31, no. 1 (2022): 287–302. doi:10.1044/2021_AJSLP-21-00110, p. 288.

13. "Serve and Return: Positive Child-Caregiver Interactions Build Strong Brains," Alberta Family Wellness, https://www.albertafamilywellness.org/what-we-know/serve-and-return#:~:text=Serve%20and%20return%20works%20like,a%20toy%20or%20a%20laugh.

14. Private email to author received February 12, 2023.
15. Ibid., 19.
16. Poole Heller, *The Power of Compassion*, 19.
17. G. C. Kaplan and M. Main, "Adult Attachment Interview Protocol," http://www.psychology.sunysb.edu/attachment/measures/content/aai_interview.pdf (accessed May 16, 2022).
18. "About the CDC-Kaiser ACE Study," U.S. Department of Health and Human Services (last updated April 6, 2021).
19. Poole Heller, *The Power of Attachment*, 59.
20. Ibid.
21. Ibid., 62
22. Ibid., 63.
23. Vedet Sar and Erdinc Ozturk, "What Is Trauma and Dissociation?," in *Trauma and Dissociation in a Cross-Cultural Perspective: Not Just a North American Phenomenon*, edited by George F. Rhodes and Vedat Sar (Binghamton: Haworth Press, 2005), 18.
24. Poole Heller, *The Power of Attachment*, 64.
25. Ibid., 67.
26. Ibid., 84.
27. Ibid., 86.
28. Main and Judith, "Discovery of an Insecure-Disorganized/Disoriented Attachment Pattern."
29. Poole Heller, *The Power of Attachment*, 122–24.
30. Ibid., 107.
31. Ibid., 109.
32. Ibid., 109–10.

4

Current Research

Elisa Monti

THE EFFECT THAT LIFE EXPERIENCES can have on one's expression and communication has fascinated scholars and practitioners for a long time. Many individuals can tell a tale from their own experience or the experience of a close person about an emotional or traumatic event changing something fundamental in their self-expression. One's voice can become "small," or "soft" as a result of grief or a painful conflict. One's voice can become tight when a painful secret is kept inside. These instances have often been observed by voice teachers, who see their students' emotions show up vocally in a number of ways.[1] This chapter is specifically intended for voice teachers and is focused on providing concise information regarding empirical and/or clinical approaches that exist in investigating how trauma can relate to the voice. Teachers of singing are often the first—sometimes the only—safe haven for students with trauma. The information provided here may hopefully add more resources in the teacher of singing's informational toolbox.

Empirical evidence about the relationship between trauma and voice still exists in limited amounts and under a handful of "categories." In light of the anecdotal and clinical interest regarding this topic, it is a mystery why the empirical component of this field is still in its infancy. This could be because effects that traumatic experiences can have on a voice become immediately apparent in cases that need immediate clinical care. These cases often involve a functional voice disorder resulting from trauma, or a case study in vocal psychotherapy of a patient utilizing vocalization to process trauma. In these cases, there is often necessity for immediate intervention and clinical care is a priority. The experimental aspects of the links between trauma and the voice become less of a primary concern. Thus, not surprisingly, much of what we know has to do with how trauma has impacted voices to levels that made them "disordered" in some way or has impacted one's expression to levels that required urgent psychotherapeutic care. In focusing on helping the individual with their immediate needs (particularly important) the curiosity for studying this phenomenon in laboratory settings is still developing.

Looking into voice function and trauma history is especially important for several reasons. Firstly, it is informative regarding care of individuals whose voice is temporarily changed or lost because of a traumatic event. Additionally, cases like these show us explicitly that some relationship exists between trauma and voice. How complex and multilayered is this relationship? What is the nature of this relationship? Can we say that trauma *causes* changes in voice or are causal components something we are just not able to claim? Why does this relationship matter even when the voice is not "disordered" or evidently changed?

Trying to answer these questions fuels the people in our field, including the writers behind this book. The road may be long, but worth every step. It is important, in this endeavor, to explore what information we currently have and the current "subcategories" it could be divided into. This is important also because our field is by nature highly interdisciplinary. In line with that, this chapter will include not only several types of evidence about the trauma-voice relationships but also additional methods that can have a therapeutic role in how traumatic experiences can influence vocal characteristics. Importantly, considerations for teachers of singing will be included as this chapter aims to be an accessory to their expertise.

Types of evidence about the trauma and voice relationship have been studied in the following:

A. Trauma and functional voice disorders
B. Empirical data on trauma history and non-disordered voices
C. Empirical data on diagnostics criteria for post-traumatic stress disorder and speech / voice indicators utilizing computational models
D. Case studies in Vocal Psychotherapy

The categories above approach different questions and utilize different methodologies. These can depend on the nature of the collected evidence and the field of study behind a specific line of questioning. For example, voice scientists sometimes approach problems differently than computational scientists in the field of psychiatry.

When it comes to general research in the relationship between voice and psychological constructs, scientists try to understand how such psychological constructs relate with vocal characteristics.[2] Across fields and studies, information can be collected in diverse ways. One component of research in the trauma field (and the voice-trauma field) is self-report measures, which involves collecting information directly from participants about their experiences. Participants answer validated questionnaires regarding whether certain categories of abuse/neglect/violence happened to them, and if so, how often. Self-report measures are sometimes frowned upon because they are not considered as rigorous as other measures; however, when it comes to collecting information about traumatic experiences, self-report can be a key component.

It is common to utilize behavioral measures, which can help tap into individuals' externalizations of inner processes[3] and bring to light the complexity of a psychological component. Importantly, researchers often employ physiological measures to provide information that cannot be obtained by observing what one says or does generally or following specific experimental instructions (e.g., utilizing a "manipulation in the laboratory").

Any study that has attempted to investigate the trauma-voice relationship has applied a combination of the methods mentioned above.

Trauma and Functional Voice Disorders

Disorders that have been described as functional (or "psychogenic" historically, as discussed in chapter 2) often present as a scenario where the patient has symptoms in the absence of structural or neurological pathology. Of note, the patient also discloses about a psychological factor or event at the onset of the voice disorder. In some cases, this psychological factor or event is considered traumatic. Cases have been documented of individuals becoming unable to produce voice after the death of a loved one, with no vocal pathology associated. Cases have also been documented of individuals whose voice quality changed drastically after an assault or extraordinarily difficult conflict.

Voice disorders that are categorized as functional can fall under several categories (e.g., dysphonia, aphonia, mutism, etc.). Describing such categories is beyond the scope of this chapter, but numerous resources exist (as mentioned in chapter 2). At the onset of functional voice disorders there can be a loss of voluntary control over phonation. The patient may be experiencing dysphonia, which is associated with various kinds of abnormal voicing, or the patient can experience aphonia, which is associated with the absence of sound. Patients can also experience sensations such as a lump in the throat, known as globus.[4]

In a study conducted by Baker and colleagues in 2013,[5] more women with psychogenic voice disorders had experienced stressful life events compared to controls. These events included traumatic events such as violent sexual assaults, serious illness, or death of loved ones in the previous twelve months.

Some of the processes underlining these mechanisms were identified as conflict over speaking out (COSO) and powerlessness in the system (PITS). COSO keeps individuals in a challenging position: knowing the negative consequences of speaking out and also living with the effects of not being able to speak out. Some experts in the field have anecdotally compared this to pressing one's foot on the gas and the brakes at the same time when driving. Communication becomes compromised in this conflict.

Another phenomenon is PITS, observed and formalized in analyses by Baker and colleagues in 2013 regarding a different layer of the speaking out issue: systemic forces. In PITS, one may choose to speak out (e.g., on racial inequality) but may feel there is little hope in doing so. This also can relate to difficulties in voicing and expressing.

In functional voice disorders, it is not unlikely for psychological and biological factors to coexist. Additionally, maladaptive personality traits and childhood trauma also tend to be present.

Empirical Data on Trauma History and Non-Disordered Voices

When it comes to more "gray" areas of voice characteristics and vocal discomfort that are not (or not yet) considered pathological, the matter of trauma and voice becomes more complex. A study conducted on singers[6] showed some initial evidence of insecure attachment style and emotional neglect history in relation to intensity measures. Measures were collected on conducting a phonetogram of the vocal range of participants and a spectrogram of a "glissando." Monti and colleagues[7] also found preliminary evidence of self-reported childhood trauma (in non-patients) linked to voice perturbation measures directly following trauma recall. Participants in this sample recorded sustained phonation on an "ah" three times before and after answering the Childhood Trauma Questionnaire. This study indicated in regression analyses that some perturbation (e.g., jitter, shimmer) variability upon trauma recall was precited by how much trauma had been reported, accounting for baseline perturbation measures. This means that some elements in the vocal signal after thinking about one's childhood were predicted by severity of trauma history reported.

Interestingly, Becker and colleagues[8] found preliminary evidence of emotional neglect in childhood being linked to the likelihood of being a "laryngoresponder," an individual who senses discomfort in the larynx as a result of experiencing stress. These findings and their future directions can be informative for all—importantly including singers—who may identify as a laryngoresponder.

Preliminary findings by Monti and colleagues also posed the question of whether some voice cues that correlate with trauma history could play a role in interpersonal violence and revictimization. Specifically, these authors have posed the question of whether vocal cues are utilized by perpetrators to target the next possible victim. Previous literature on body language[9] points to perpetrator's ability to read elements others may not be able to. This also would point to a relationship between trauma and voice, with possible social implications.

Empirical Data on Diagnostics Criteria for Post-Traumatic Stress Disorder and Speech / Voice Indicators Utilizing Computational Models

The subfield of computational science in voice and trauma is opening fascinating doors.

Marmar and colleagues[10] conducted a study on speech markers for post-traumatic stress disorder in U.S. veterans. Marmar et al. investigated the potential of utilizing speech and voice markers diagnostically as it could facilitate some of the challenges in diagnosing PTSD. This can include clinical biases, the need for more objective measures, as well as addressing the difficulty patients have with disclosing traumatic experiences and their symptoms.

Several studies have pointed to biological markers of PTSD including alterations in neural structures and circuit functioning, genomics, neurochemistry, immune functioning, and psychophysiology. Studying voice could serve as a new and noninvasive indicator to be added to other diagnostic tools. American warzone-exposed male Iraq and Afghanistan veterans, with no depression, no psychosis, and no history of recent or current trauma were clinically interviewed. Acoustic features were extracted from small frames in the voice signal. The Random Forest probability algorithm was used to build a classifier function using speech markers to predict PTSD. Compared to controls, participants with PTSD presented with more monotonous, less varying tonality, more monotonous speech segments, more occurrence of slow speech production, flatter speech, less animated speech, flatter speech with less energy activation.

Previous literature in this subfield includes evidence collected by Van den Broek, Van der Sluis, and Dijkstra[11] who asked individuals with PTSD to speak two different types of narratives and found that numerous voice indicators (related to frequency, energy, and amplitude) of speech accounted for or related to stress symptoms. Also, Scherer and colleagues[12] found that in response to positive, negative, and neutral interview prompts, those with PTSD exhibited differences in acoustic cues in voice and decreased vowel space when speaking.[13] These findings indicate that some voice acoustic features could differ in individuals who not only have a history of trauma, but also who have symptomatology consistent with PTSD.

Case Studies in Vocal Psychotherapy

Vocal psychotherapy is a voice-based model of music therapy. Vocal psychotherapy is also a trauma-based type of clinical intervention. It involves the use of breath, natural sounds, vocal improvisation, and songs. These tools are a fundamental part of the healing process and growth of the client in the vocal psychotherapy philosophy. This model, created by Diane Austin, is based on the notion that the voice is the primary instrument.[14] Also, techniques such as *vocal holding* and *free associative singing* are core practices in vocal psychotherapy. Vocal holding involves the use of two chords chosen by the client and played by the therapist. The client is invited to begin vocalizing in a way that feels natural for them, and the therapist accompanies them vocally in ways that are also representative of developmental stages (for example, unison can be seen as symbiosis, a lower harmony can be seen as grounding, echoing can be seen as mirroring). This musical environment aims at creating a reparative experience for the client so that they can feel safer and freer while exploring their own emotions and states. Free associative singing begins in a similar way but evolves into the use of words, and the therapist repeats and sometimes reframes a lot of what the client sings using an eye for dabbling, similar to techniques and psychodrama.

Some of the biggest lessons that can be taken from case studies in vocal psychotherapy are that clients come into the room with specific vocal cues that anecdotally seem to relate to difficult traumatic histories and evolve into something different during the course of the therapy. The clients are instructed to utilize their voice as part of the therapeutic process, but they are never instructed to target a specific sound or to place their voice in a particular way. Therefore, we can safely say that the changes that occur come from a psychotherapeutic approach, not a vocal approach. The evidence that comes from case studies in vocal psychotherapy is purely anecdotal, but similar to some cases of functional voice disorders; the connections between the trauma history, the vocal cues, and the vocal changes after the therapeutic approach was conducted, seem to point to a relationship.

Additional Related Methods

Eye Movement Desensitization and Reprocessing (EMDR) is a form of psychotherapy that has been empirically validated in the treatment of posttraumatic stress disorder and other types of conditions. EMDR was introduced in 1989 with the publication of a randomized controlled trial evaluating its effects on victims of trauma. EMDR therapy occurs in eight phases of treatment, involving elements such as history taking, preparation, assessment, desensitization, installation, body scan, enclosure, and reassessment.

Describing these phases in detail is beyond the scope of this chapter, but some components of these phases include procedures such as identifying the events that have brought the individual to the current state, what triggers and needs of the client need to be evaluated. The client becomes educated on symptoms and techniques that foster stabilization and a sense of personal control. During the assessment phase, the client is asked to access the image or negative belief currently held and the desired positive belief, current emotion, and physical sensations. The sensitization phase incorporates eye movements (sometimes taps or tones) that allow the spontaneous emergence of insights, emotions, physical sensations, and other memories. Importantly, the installation phase enhances the validity of the new positive affect and beliefs.[15]

The Montello Method for Performance Wellness

The Montello Method for Performance Wellness and the subsequent nonprofit organization Performance Wellness, INC, were created by Dr. Louise Montello between the late 1980s and the early 1990s. Dr. Montello's mission was to foster transformation for creatives, performers, musicians, and artists through the healing power of music and creativity (also including yoga and behavioral medicine). Performance Wellness is a proactive approach where the musician or artist themselves learn to utilize music and art as a source of healing. When they have lost the passion or joy for their craft or instrument, Performance Wellness helps them understand what happened and how, and how to return to the original state of joy in creative endeavors. Addressing problems such as performance anxiety, perfectionism, performance-related trauma, developmental trauma, creative blocks, and more Performance Wellness helps restore an artist's passion.

KATMAN Technique

The KATMAN technique is a brain-based healing technique developed to help individuals who suffer from autonomic dysfunction and tension of the dura, the outer layer of tissue that protects the brain. A number of conditions can contribute to such problems including PTSD or complex-PTSD, postural orthostatic tachycardia syndrome (POTS), COVID-19 and long-COVID syndrome, and other types of conditions associated with autonomic nervous system problems.

The KATMAN technique works to stimulate vagal tone and improve neurologic function. It was developed by two doctors of chiropractic, Dr. Manuel

Marco Mazzini and Dr. Katinka van der Merwe. Their collaborative observations and techniques were developed while working with some serious cases of neurologic dysfunction, often associated with acute or chronic trauma. The KATMAN technique shares some principles with the well-known polyvagal theory, mentioned in chapter 2.

How Does This Inform Voice Teaching?

The laboratory evaluated empirical evidence around these techniques is sometimes lacking, but all the mentioned techniques have demonstrated through numerous case studies that a substantial number of patients can highly benefit from these methods. These case studies described in the literature of each technique have often included singers. How these methodologies can positively affect the voice can potentially happen via numerous ways, somatic, neurologic (and autonomic), psychodynamic, cognitive, and more (and often through various combinations and overlaps). The coming years may see different empirical approaches take place in studying the mentioned methods.

The purpose in describing the empirical findings around the voice-trauma relationship and methodologies that therapeutically address this relationship can be informative for voice teachers in several ways. One element is that it can be informative and empowering to keep in mind that what happens vocally for singers who have been through trauma is now finally starting to become an interest of research. In terms of empirical findings, it is good to be conservative and not see your specific student in the results of a study. Nonetheless, studies include real people with real experiences, and a set of findings may be closer to the inner workings of a specific voice student than we might know. For example, Monti et al.[16] discuss an inverse correlation between a singer's insecure attachment and their maximum loudness. This may induce one to think, "Oh, my, I clearly exhibit traits of anxious attachment style, what if my loudness is strongly or even permanently affected?" It is important to keep in mind that this study speaks primarily about the participants who were in it; how these findings generalize to the "singing general population" is as always one of the difficult questions in science. Also, the study does not speak of *causation* at all, so it does not claim that insecure attachment "causes" lower maximum loudness.

How does this speak of my specific student? It may or may not but keeping these data in mind helps the voice teacher approach all "loudness" related matters with an even broader array of possibilities, knowing that among the known variables that may relate to one's loudness, anxious attachment may be one as well. Having empirical evidence in one's back pocket can add to their perspective.

Notes

1. Diane Austin, *The Theory and Practice of Vocal Psychotherapy: Songs of the Self* (Jessica Kingsley Publishers, 2009).

2. M. Van Mersbergen, "Research Approaches in the Intersection of Voice Disorders and Psychology," in *Psychology of Voice Disorders*, by R. Sataloff, D. Rosen, and J. Sataloff, second edition (Plural Publishing, 2020).

3. Ibid.

4. Deborah Caputo Rosen, Johnathan Brandon Sataloff, and Robert Thayer Sataloff, *Psychology of Voice Disorders* (Plural Publishing, 2020).

5. Janet Baker, David Ben-Tovim, Andrew Butcher, Adrian Esterman, and Kristin McLaughlin, "Psychosocial Risk Factors Which May Differentiate between Women with Functional Voice Disorder, Organic Voice Disorder and a Control Group," *International Journal of Speech-Language Pathology* 15, no. 6 (2013): 547–63.

6. Elisa Monti, David C. Kidd, Linda M. Carroll, and Emanuele Castano, "What's in a Singer's Voice: The Effect of Attachment, Emotions and Trauma," *Logopedics Phoniatrics Vocology* 42, no. 2 (2017): 62–72.

7. Elisa Monti, Wendy D'Andrea, Steven Freed, David C. Kidd, Shelley Feuer, Linda M. Carroll, and Emanuele Castano, "Does Self-Reported Childhood Trauma Relate to Vocal Acoustic Measures? Preliminary Findings at Trauma Recall," *Journal of Nonverbal Behavior* 45, no. 3 (2021): 389–408.

8. Diana Rose Becker, Brett Welch, Elisa Monti, Harmony Sullivan, and Leah B. Helou, "Investigating Past Trauma in Laryngoresponders versus Non-Laryngoresponders: Piloting New Methods in an Exploratory Study," *Journal of Voice* (2022).

9. Sarah Wheeler, "The Convergence of Psychopathy, Self-Rated Vulnerability, and Other-Rated Vulnerability" (thesis, Brock University, St. Catharines, 2011).

10. Charles R. Marmar, Adam D. Brown, Meng Qian, Eugene Laska, Carole Siegel, Meng Li, Duna Abu-Amara et al., "Speech-Based Markers for Posttraumatic Stress Disorder in US Veterans," *Depression and Anxiety* 36, no. 7 (2019): 607–16.

11. E. L. Van den Broek, F. Van der Sluis, and T. Dijkstra, "Telling the Story and Re-Living the Past: How Speech Analysis Can Reveal Emotions in Post-Traumatic Stress Disorder (PTSD) Patients," in *Sensing Emotions*, edited by J. Westerink, M. Krans, and M. Ouwerkerk, Philips Research Book Series, vol 12 (Dordrecht: Springer, 2010), 153–80, https://doi.org/10.1007/978-90-481-3258-4_10.

12. Stefan Scherer, Giota Stratou, Jonathan Gratch, and Louis-Philippe Morency, "Investigating Voice Quality as a Speaker-Independent Indicator of Depression and PTSD," in Interspeech (conference, August 2013), 847–51.

13. Stefan Scherer, Gale M. Lucas, Jonathan Gratch, Albert Skip Rizzo, and Louis-Philippe Morency, "Self-Reported Symptoms of Depression and PTSD Are Associated with Reduced Vowel Space in Screening Interviews," *IEEE Transactions on Affective Computing* 7, no. 1 (2015): 59–73.

14. Austin, *The Theory and Practice of Vocal Psychotherapy*.

15. Francine Shapiro, "The Role of Eye Movement Desensitization and Reprocessing (EMDR) Therapy in Medicine: Addressing the Psychological and Physical Symptoms Stemming from Adverse Life Experiences," *The Permanente Journal* 18, no. 1 (2014): 71.

16. Monti et al., "What's in a Singer's Voice," 62–72.

II
THE ROLE OF THE VOICE PRACTITIONER

5

Singing in Co-Harmony

An Introduction to Trauma-Informed Voice Care

Megan Durham

[A note from the author: I acknowledge how my multiple privileges—including race, class, education, access, gender identity, and ability—impact the lens with which I approach this work. I also acknowledge both my experience and imperfection with this material, honoring my scope of practice as a voice professional, not a mental healthcare provider. There is no discussion of grief, disconnection, and trauma that will land in the same way for every body. This work is constantly adapting to new research and terminology based on shifts in the landscape of social justice and mental health. Two things can be true: there are rarely "right" answers when working in human complexity AND we can offer informed, compassionate care to the best of our ability.]

SARA WAS A FIFTY-YEAR-OLD PROFESSIONAL SINGER whose teenage son passed away five years before I met her. Immense grief manifested physically throughout her body as chronic fatigue, intrusive thoughts, emotional and physical numbness, muscle tension dysphonia, and disordered breathing (hyperventilation). When we first started working together, she would tearfully exclaim, "I can't access my low breath, and when I do, I feel too much!" For several years after her son's passing, Sara's lifelong breath for singing—in the lower abdomen—triggered feelings of overwhelm, intense grief, and constriction. Feeling shame over not being able to "breathe correctly" (her words—having been told by a voice professional that if she could not breathe properly, she would never regain "healthy vocal function") exacerbated this emotional distress. Sara's body was habitually mobilized for threat, armoring her against further emotional pain. This made diaphragmatic breathing feel unattainable and emotionally untethered.

After anchoring to the present moment with mindful movement, Sara described the sensations that were uncomfortable. She pointed to her abdomen, using words like rigid, gut-wrenching, and suffocating. After spending a few moments sitting with these feelings, I asked Sara where she would like to feel her breath. Was there anywhere in the body that felt secure, like "home"? She pointed to her heart center and around her back between the shoulder blades. Sara seemed surprised and relieved to find that this space was available to her. Words like whole, spacious, intentional came to her mind, as well as soothing images from nature. In that moment, breathing through her nose and into her heart center allowed for present moment connection. With this breath, her voice soared. In time, Sara began remembering other spaces in her body that had once seemed separate, and her breath deepened on its own.

When you work with bodies, it is highly likely that you interface with the complexities of chronic stress or trauma. In fact, a current statistic indicates that it is more likely that an individual walking into a voice studio or clinic has experienced abuse or neglect than it is for them to be left-handed. Distressing circumstances and compound stress, whether experienced at once or over a period of time, can result in posttraumatic stress.[1] The biopsychosocial effects of traumatic stress can inhibit vocal function and create communication difficulty, voice loss, fear of speaking, performance anxiety, and a feeling of being silenced. Others may struggle with trauma resulting from oppressive systems like racism, classism, ableism, heterosexism, and colonialism (among countless others) that frequently prevent access to basic needs, let alone mental healthcare resources.

As voice professionals, we can acknowledge how traumatic stress impacts voices, and offer embodied, compassionate tools that promote nervous system support for both ourselves and our students—all while maintaining our scope of practice. Trauma-informed voice care (TIVC) recognizes the profound neurological, physiological, psychological, and social impacts that trauma can have on singing bodies. By cultivating mindfulness, present-moment orientation, self-inquiry, and an emphasis on observation rather than correction, TIVC provides a collaborative approach to voice work that empowers individuals to identify their innate creative agency more clearly.

This chapter provides an overview of how trauma can impact the individuals that we work with, summarizing and reviewing information from part 1, and offers strategies for creating a supportive environment within the context of voice care. Trauma-informed voice professionals aim to cultivate a supportive presence that can mindfully and imperfectly navigate both comfort and discomfort. We can begin this process by noticing our own physical and emotional sensations and engaging in co-regulation (or co-harmony)[2]—establishing compassionate, nonjudgmental reciprocal connections. By acknowledging how trauma and chronic stress can manifest in our bodies, we learn to hold more informed spaces for individuals to communicate with more ease, creativity, and authenticity.

What Is Trauma?

Neuroscientist and researcher Dr. Stephen Porges often says that trauma is a chronic disruption of connectedness.[3] Author and activist Staci Haines elaborates:

> "Trauma is an experience, series of experiences, and/or impacts from social conditions that break or betray our inherent need for safety, belonging, and dignity. They . . . result in us having to vie between these inherent needs, often setting one against the other."[4] For example, it might leave us with the impact of "I can be safe but not connected (isolated), or "I have to give up my dignity to be safe or connected."[4]

At our core, we yearn for community. In times of distress, the necessity to protect ourselves overrides our need to connect with others. Trauma can occur when we are unable to feel safe in our environments, in our bodies, in our families, or in our communities, and the impact of this stress outweighs our ability to access supportive resources. It is important to emphasize that not everything that is difficult or disconnecting is traumatic. The words *trauma*, *traumatized*, and *triggered* are often trivialized and marketed (particularly in social media spaces) as what is colloquially referred to as "Instagram therapy." Our bodies can exhibit various physiological and psychological responses to threatening or painful situations without manifesting as posttraumatic stress.

As discussed in chapter 1, much trauma research has been dedicated to how the autonomic nervous system (ANS) responds to external cues of safety and danger. Comprised of the sympathetic (SNS) and parasympathetic branches (PNS), the ANS is the primary regulating system for the body's many functions, including heart rate, digestion, respiration rate, elimination, and sexual arousal. However, the human body is not as cleanly categorized as this definition of the ANS might suggest. In fact, the autonomic space model created by Berntson et. al. in 1991[5] suggests that there are nine possible states (including blended) that our ANS may be in, and that the SNS and PNS are not "universally reciprocal"—meaning, when one turns on, the other doesn't necessarily shut down. Rather, we can have a variety of states that respond to the complexities and challenges of being human. The ANS and its connection to our bodies and voices is far more intricate than a linear spectrum from calm to anxious. The following is an attempt to provide a bit of clarity to a vastly dynamic, interconnected system—humans (voices) cannot be reduced to models of behavior.

The SNS provides us with survival energy, mobilizing the body's vital resources for daily functional tasks. When hyper-aroused due to immediate or perceived threat, the SNS shifts into "fight or flight" mode, characterized by increased heart rate, the release of adrenaline and cortisol, muscle contraction (including the diaphragm, which stabilizes the core muscles as they activate to "run"), rapid breathing, and sweaty palms. As the body prepares to flee from danger, we may experience feelings of overwhelm, hyperarousal, anxiety, anger, and hypervigilance. A singer in this state may not be able to access a "low breath" because the diaphragm is preparing for defense, not for Debussy. In these moments, it is important to be mindful that the impact of pedagogical cues like "just relax" or "breathe deeply" can bypass the singer's current emotional and physiological experience, creating more stress. The body is doing exactly what it was designed to do—find a safer alternative.

In contrast, the parasympathetic nervous system (PNS) is associated with the common phrase "rest and digest." Signaling well-being and groundedness, the PNS can help us to feel at home in our bodies, connected to ourselves and those around us. It should be noted that a resourced nervous system is not calm all the time—it is adaptable, ready for mobilization, and able to ride the natural waves of mood and energy fluctuation.[6] After all, transformation, creativity, and purpose necessitate stimulation in some form—artistry requires activation. In moments of hypo-arousal, however, we may experience feelings of separation, numbness, depression, reduced movement capacity or futility. The cycle between fight, flight, freeze, and connection keeps us alive and able to make choices about which people or activities make us feel connected and which signal danger.[7] Often referred to as neuroception, this decision about who and what feels safe is out of our conscious control—perhaps a "gut feeling" emerges. Researcher Stephen Porges writes,

> The nervous system, through the processing of sensory information from the environment and from the viscera, continuously evaluates risk. Since the neural evaluation of risk does not require conscious awareness and may involve subcortical limbic structures, the term neuroception was introduced to emphasize a neural process, distinct from perception, that is capable of distinguishing environmental (and visceral) features that are safe, dangerous, or life-threatening.[8]

When intense situations prevent us from making choices about how to respond to cues of danger, we may feel trapped in either fight, flight, or freeze responses (or a combination), long after the initial event has passed. This sense of immobility, hopelessness, or constant hypervigilance can take hold in the body as trauma.

Trauma can manifest differently in every body. While we might tend to think of trauma as a response to a singular event, therapist Resmaa Menekem explains that

> trauma can also be the body's response to a long sequence of smaller wounds. It can be a response to anything that is experienced as too much, too soon, or too fast. Trauma can also be the body's response to anything unfamiliar or anything

it doesn't understand, even if it isn't cognitively dangerous. The body doesn't reason; it's hardwired to protect itself and react to sensation and movement.[9]

Trauma is not the event itself; it is how our nervous system responds to the event and can result from any event that we perceive to be beyond our threshold for autonomous, embodied, and instinctive response. Much like an animal "shakes off" unwanted experiences, humans require physical and emotional movement to process traumatic events. Author and therapist, Peter Levine, explains:

> A threatened human must discharge all of the energy mobilized to negotiate that threat, or it will become a victim of trauma. This residual energy does not simply go away. It persists in the body, and often forces the formation of a wide variety of symptoms (anxiety, depression, psychosomatic and behavioral problems). These symptoms are the organism's way of containing the undischarged residual energy.[10]

Trauma can occur after any event in which an individual does not have the time or choice to complete this natural survival cycle. If an individual is not allowed or empowered to naturally discharge an experience of sexual assault, abuse, bullying, domestic violence, neglect, community violence, racism, emotional abuse, car accident, forced displacement, war, natural disaster, terrorism, a medical illness or procedure, arrest or incarceration, emotional manipulation/abuse, separation from family, collective disaster (e.g., a pandemic), or historical trauma, they may experience long-lasting impacts of trauma in the body.[11]

While the physical and mental effects of trauma can vary widely and are highly complex, common indications include anxiety, depression, insomnia, flashbacks, numbness, clenched muscles (neck, shoulders, jaw, tongue, diaphragm), sunken chest (heavy heart), hypervigilance, disregulated breathing, and an absence of agency/powerlessness.[12] Any one of these presentations can significantly impact vocal function. An emerging research field, the intersection of trauma and voice, reveals that our lived experiences impact the efficacy and authenticity of our spoken (and sung) communication. One study, conducted by Helou, Rosen, Wang, and Verdollini Abbott, found that stressful circumstances notably increase activity in the intrinsic laryngeal muscles.[13] Researcher and psychotherapist Elisa Monti elaborates that traumatic stress can result in significant vocal difficulty, including psychogenic dysphonia:

> This is a type of voice disorder that generally occurs in the absence of laryngeal pathology and can be comorbid with a type of psychological disorder or traumatic event (or both) that interferes with voice control. . . . [T]here are multiple ways in which a traumatic experience can have effects on the voice. Voice physiology, acoustics, and perceptual components are altered by the physiology of the rest of the body, which is itself influenced by emotions.[14]

As noted in chapter 4, another groundbreaking study conducted in 2019 at the NYU School of Medicine investigated the subtle speech patterns of PTSD patients. The authors found the following:

> Patients with PTSD tended to speak in flatter speech, with less articulation of the tongue and lips and a more monotonous tone, the researchers reported. . . . We thought the telling features would reflect agitated speech. In point of fact, when we saw the data, the features are flatter, more atonal speech. We were capturing the numbness that is so typical of PTSD patients. . . . We've known for a long time that you can tell how someone is doing from their voice.[15]

Although the acute and long-term effects of trauma on the voice are in the early stages of research, possible physiological responses associated with depression, anxiety, and/or trauma might include intense shame, fear, or discomfort with communication, including voice loss; feeling overwhelmed by tasks; difficulty sensing movement, breath, or vibration inside the body (interoception); overactive SNS responses like shaking, sweating, gasping for breath, nausea, and so forth during lessons or performances; "freeze" response in lessons or on stage (PNS/dorsal branch).

Directly or indirectly, singers can feel stigmatized for the ways in which their bodies have protected them during threatening experiences in the past—such as gasping for air or difficulty exhaling consistently. Often, these are habituated, involuntary nervous system responses created in moments of stress to armor the body against danger (e.g., the diaphragm acting as a core stabilizer, preparing to fight or flee). It is critical to point out that these responses are not necessarily due to trauma—our bodies' responses to danger are normal, healthy, and biologically intelligent! The paradox of trauma-informed care is that we are not assuming that the responses we observe are "trauma"; and yet, we can reframe how we interact with all singing bodies, treating any response with dignity and reverence. How does it change the way we think about voice pedagogy when we consider that many responses historically labeled "vocal faults" are in fact survival strategies? Instead of treating these responses as "problems," let us honor how the body has functioned as a fortress in times of distress. Singers should not be made to feel that their bodies' natural responses to stress are incorrect, inappropriate, or render them "unhealthy" singers or "ineffective" performers.

It is also necessary to examine how ableism influences how we decide what "healthy, balanced, beautiful" looks and sounds like. In her seminal work, *The Body Is Not an Apology: The Power of Radical Self Love*, author and activist Sonya Renee Taylor writes, "There is no standard of health that is achievable for all bodies. Our belief that there should be anchors the systematic oppression of ableism, and reinforces the notion that people with illnesses and disabilities have defective bodies rather than different bodies."[16] How might voice professionals hear this message within the context of the singing body? What happens when we exchange the word "bodies" for "voices?" Does this message challenge constructs about voice pedagogy?

Becca's Story

Becca was a reading specialist who loved to sing avocationally in her church choir. Although singing had always been a source of healing, she had recently experienced total voice loss when a stressful experience triggered a memory of childhood sexual abuse. Although slowly regaining vocal function, Becca felt intense shame and fear when singing, and was inundated with intrusive thoughts that if she could not be "accurate," her voice would not be acceptable. Cues like "you're not breathing correctly, take a deeper breath" from a well-meaning choir director exacerbated these feelings. Gasping for more air through the mouth activated her fight or flight instincts and caused hyperventilation. Becca was inhaling more oxygen than her body could metabolize, thinking that more air meant better singing. Our bodies only use 25 percent of the oxygen that we inhale, and we need a residual amount of carbon dioxide for optimal functioning. Carbon dioxide is a necessary hormone that regulates blood flow, airflow, and our mood. When we deplete the body of this natural resource by taking in too much oxygen, anxiety increases.[17] With habitual patterns like "deep breathing" through the mouth, Becca's vocal onset was breathy and hesitant, creating a sound quality that she felt was inauthentic. The cycle of fear, hyperventilation, phonation, and shame was a deeply ingrained pattern.

Within ten minutes of steady, natural breaths in through the nose, Becca's demeanor shifted. She reported feeling grounded, less tense, and less focused on accuracy. Her instinct to "protect" her sound softened. Further, when we isolated inhalation to the left nostril (activating the PNS),[18] Becca's vocal on set was immediately clear and connected, and a vibrant, warm, authentic timbre emerged. Becca did not need to learn how to breathe; she needed to remind herself that she already knew how. We gently invited the muscles of protection to rest, as they were not required in this moment.

Trauma-Informed Practice

Singers like Becca often feel stuck in patterns of how the body and voice "should" feel based on other's suggestions or subjective sound ideals, rather than trusting their own instincts. Instructing a singer how or what to feel in their body may not acknowledge their present moment or their lived experience. Perhaps their breath is shallow because a lower breath feels inaccessible or unsafe. For some survivors, breath itself is triggering. We must take care that our language does not prioritize the teacher's goal over the student's body. Instead, invitation-based language (e.g., asking "Where does this land? What sensations are arising for you?") grants permission for the singer to experience breath and spaciousness in any location—the shoulders, clavicle, pelvis, throat, thoracic spine, sinuses, toes, and so on! We can encourage singers to observe sensations and movement possibilities without judgment or enforcing normative conditions for how singing bodies should inhabit space. A starting point for empowering our students to reclaim this kind of vocal dignity is to understand the basic foundations of trauma-informed practice.

What Does "Trauma-Informed" Mean?

According to the CDC's Substance Abuse and Mental Health Services Administration, the phrase "trauma-informed' is comprised of six principles:[19]

- *Safety*: Ensuring that people feel physically and psychologically safe or grounded, both with the practitioner and in the space itself.
- *Trust*: The practitioner conducts themselves with the utmost transparency, with the goal of gaining and maintaining trust with the client.
- *Peer Support*: "Peer support [meaning other survivors/individuals who have experienced trauma] and mutual self-help are key vehicles for establishing safety and hope, building trust, enhancing collaboration, and utilizing their stories and lived experience to promote recovery and healing."[20]
- *Collaboration*: The practitioner creates an environment of mutual respect, dialog, and collaborative decision making.
- *Empowerment, Voice, and Choice*: The practitioner honors the individual's lived experience and cultivates an environment of agency, choice, and self-efficacy. Practitioners "understand the importance of power differentials and ways in which clients, historically, have been diminished in voice and choice and are often recipients of coercive treatment."[21]
- *Cultural, Historical, and Gender Issues*: The practitioner "moves past cultural stereotypes and biases (e.g., based on race, ethnicity, sexual orientation, age, religion, gender- identity, geography, etc.); offers access to gender responsive services; leverages the healing value of traditional cultural connections; incorporates policies, protocols, and processes that are responsive to the racial, ethnic and cultural needs of individuals served; and recognizes and addresses historical trauma."[22]

The trauma-informed journey is a life-long, unequivocal commitment to social justice, decolonization, cultural humility, and anti-oppression in its many forms. We'll continue discussion on implementing these principles in chapter 6.

When seeking to establish these principles, we can never assume what "safety" feels like in another body or that we can provide it. We can create considered spaces of inquiry, creativity, choice, and challenge (when appropriate); however, creating a "safe space" should not assume that what feels safe for us creates safety for someone else. Our sense of well-being is relative to our lived experience. As teachers, we can provide tools like mindful movement, nose breathing, meditation, and other forms of physical and mental sensing that promote embodied safety in a considered environment. Perhaps most importantly, we can be sure that the space itself is filled with choice: the lighting, the temperature, a visible exit, a thoughtful use of props, repertoire, inclusive and affirming language, and even the process of sound-making. In the words of intimacy director, sexological bodyworker, and creator of the Wheel of Consent, Betty Martin, the choosing is more important than the doing.[23]

Each of these six components serves to rebuild a sense of empowerment, trust, and hope in the individual; however, in truth, there is no "arrival" at being trauma informed. Although these principles provide a scaffolding, working with trauma is a nonlinear journey of creating compassionate spaces for messy learning. It is acknowledging multiple truths about our body—I have an injury, and I am resilient; our mind—I experience depression, and I am powerful; and our voice—I feel afraid to sing, and my voice has agency. As a trauma-informed voice teacher, each student provides a new opportunity to learn, to stumble, to apologize when harm has been done, and perhaps most importantly, to do our own work of self-realization and accountability.

Another significant piece of trauma-informed awareness involves recognizing our position of power (especially those who identify as white, cisgender, and/or heterosexual). The lineage of Western classical voice pedagogy often establishes a "master/apprentice" binary, where the teacher/practitioner assumes full control and knowledge of the student's voice (and body).[24] This control may be subtle: "I want you to feel it here . . . " "You're not doing it correctly . . . "; or more overt: unwanted/unannounced touching, shame-based motivation, and even abuse. We must actively consider how voice pedagogy is rooted in Eurocentric aesthetic ideals and examine if our opinions and actions reflect the bias of oppressive systems. In the text, *Humane Music Education for the Common Good*, contributing author Emily Good-Perkins writes,

> Historically, bel canto singing was intertwined with colonialism. In 19th century Britain, vocal pedagogy was referred to as "voice culture," where "culture" in the 19th century was synonymous with "civilization." The "othering" of singing

voices justified the use of vocal teaching to "civilize" and refine those who were not part of white bourgeois culture for the betterment of society . . . voice culture provided the opportunity for re-forming the voice, for colonizing yet more of the other's body . . . the singing voice . . . became the vehicle for "symbolic violence."[25]

Trauma-informed care unambiguously asserts that no one is in charge of the student's voice/body but the student. Understanding this critical boundary helps teachers to cultivate mindful, rational leadership. In his book *To Have or To Be*, humanist philosopher Erich Fromm writes, "Rational authority is based on competence, and it helps the person who leans on it to grow. Irrational authority is based on power and serves to exploit the person subjected to it."[26] Becoming aware of our position of power, the biases that often come with this power, and the responsibility that we have to our students to maintain our own learning, competency, and humility builds rational authority in the voice studio. Leading with integrity allows us to move beyond making assumptions about our students' preferences and abilities based solely on gender, race, culture, body, or sexuality. We can instead invite singers to explore choices that feel authentic to their lived experiences and limitless creative potential.

The power-over dynamic described by Fromm can sometimes take the form of a "rescuer" persona, underscored by the age-old trope: voice lessons are like therapy/my voice teacher is my therapist. This is a complicated topic filled with both/and. There is an undeniable, innate "healing" power in music and sound making—not to mention the significant impact (both conscious and unconscious) that interpersonal connection (co-harmony) can have in the healing process. Studies in neurobiology, music therapy, psychotherapy, and countless other disciplines have proven that sound builds neuroplasticity, resiliency, and present-moment orientation. Additionally, voice teachers can approach the therapeutic benefit of singing, co-creation, and artistic expression with great humility for their potency, especially as most of us are not trained psychotherapists.

The "voice teacher as healer/therapist" analogy can become problematic when we frequently position ourselves as the source of the healing, crossing the scope of practice boundary and assuming a role that we are not equipped to handle. As we'll discuss in greater depth in chapter 6, training in trauma work, somatics, yoga, nervous system support, and so on does not give us permission to make psychological and psycho-physiological assumptions about singers. Further, psychological tools and interventions cannot be decontextualized, reduced, and repackaged as workshop gimmicks, quick fixes, or body hacks in the name of "deepening artistic expression" or "accessing the true creative self." This includes pushing students to the edge of emotional catharsis in repertoire or character work without having any training or supportive scaffolding to hold what might emerge. Our unconscious material is vast and working with emotional and physical reactivity is an intricate and sacred endeavor.

We could ask, who am I continually centering as the conduit of this "therapeutic work": the music and sound itself, or me, the teacher/practitioner? What do we mean by therapy/therapeutic, and what is my impact (not just intention) in the space? Is there an understood, consensual agreement about how this space functions? Are there mutual expectations for what happens in the space, and why is the singer here? Am I taking on a "healer," "rescuer," or "savior" persona, wherein I frequently impart emotional and psychological wisdom to my student, especially in an attempt to keep them coming back?

As we seek to create and honor our own scope of practice as voice teachers, we must be in a constant relationship with knowing and unknowing, what we offer and what we do not. Recognizing that the voice studio is a place of powerful conscious and unconscious connection, we can affirm that our boundaries are as sacred as our offerings, and it is not our role to "save" voices.

Singing in Co-Harmony

We have a biological imperative to connect. When we co-regulate (or co-harmonize), we support one another by cultivating trust, reciprocity, and the kind of healthy boundaries previously mentioned. In her book *The Polyvagal Theory in Therapy: Engaging the Rhythm of Regulation*, Deb Dana tells us, "Co regulation [or co-harmony] creates a physiological platform of safety that supports a psychological story of security that leads to social engagement. The autonomic nervous systems of two individuals find sanctuary in a co-created experience of connection."[27] In states of distress or distraction, teachers cannot clearly communicate information, and our students may not be able to receive new information. One way that we can help to deactivate this "alert" response is to acknowledge (mindfully or verbally) what is happening right now. The most important resource that we can provide our students is our intentional presence and language that clearly communicates I am here, help me understand—especially in times of discomfort or awkwardness. This framework supports subsequent learning and information processing, building a compassionate bridge between intentions and actions.

As teachers, we can notice when our own bodies feel grounded, disconnected, or activated so that we can be a more effective co-harmonizer for our students. When we build self-awareness, it becomes easier to attune to our students' needs. We can more clearly sense when it's time for challenge or time for rest, time to integrate or time to compartmentalize. Being present allows us to pause and ask, what is necessary in this moment—my guidance, or my patience? More information, or more space? It may be challenging to answer these questions in the moment, and we have to rest more in the asking than the answering. We'll discuss tools for the teacher in chapter 8.

Part of our role as a co-harmonizer asks that we sit with discomfort, the insecurity of not knowing, and be willing to pivot, evolve, and unlearn. In fact, by the time you read this article, it is likely that I will have adopted different language around these concepts and gained new insight based on current research. Honoring the present moment means continually embodying humility and checking one's own assumptions. It's easy to revel in the moments of discovery from students, but the "I'm still discouraged" moments can make us feel uncomfortable, often defensive of our strategy, approach, or track record. Let us take care that our impulse "to prove" does not invalidate the student's frustration, becoming more about our need to fix, to please, to perform, than the student's need to be heard. When we stay attuned to the student's physical and emotional cues in moments of disappointment, as well as our own internal responses, we can step back, take a breath, and create space between our feelings (I feel defensive!) and our actions (yet, I can respond with compassion).

Resisting immediate change, sitting with discomfort, or being willing to think outside of the "(any genre) voice pedagogy box" are critical aspects to honoring our students' lived experiences. In Sara's case, it was more important for her to feel more safely embodied with a breath of her choice than for me to ask her to connect to a place that felt inaccessible, though more traditional. It was necessary for her to articulate her sensation, receive validation, and make collaborative choices about how to proceed. Cultivating a co-harmonic presence helps us to provide a space for processing conflict, especially when evidence-based vocal techniques may not be beneficial in the moment. By validating the student's concerns, we communicate that it is possible to sit with doubt and also recognize wholeness. In this way, we can help students to learn that they can hold multiple truths about their voices and experiences—I am learning, this is challenging, *and* I am resilient; I can ask difficult questions.

When we as teachers are not aware of our own current physical and emotional states, these choices become more difficult. Our self-limiting beliefs, feelings of threat, or defensiveness can creep into the space. If you feel these armoring tendencies arise, pause and ask, do my internal sensations and subsequent actions reflect an environment of trust, choice, and collaboration, or hesitation, power, and resistance? In the latter case, can I respond to myself as a self-compassionate witness rather than a judge, tenderly affirming that this reaction is human? I can both take responsibility and affirm that I am worthy, even when I am not able to be present in the ways that I intend.

Embodying a Supportive Presence

Our nervous systems are designed to naturally cycle through periods of activity, mobilization, rest, and inertia. Under traumatic stress, it is overwhelming to negotiate this process when we feel disconnected from our body and our surroundings, and do not have the resources to ride the waves of this cycle. Because trauma makes it difficult to trust our external and internal experiences, embodiment practices help individuals regain present-moment awareness. Jungian Somatics creator, Jane Clapp, defines embodiment as "to provide with a body; incarnate; make corporeal: to embody a spirit. Embodiment can simply mean living in conscious awareness of our body in whatever way is available to any given body at any given moment in time."[28] Cultivating this conscious awareness takes time and is often nonlinear. It is also inherently tied to our relationship with the land and environment, as colonization has disconnected us from our roots, our sense of the ground, and our responsibility to be in a sustainable relationship with the collective body.

One way to practice conscious "embodiment" is through developing awareness of *exteroception*, what is happening outside of my body (e.g., I feel my feet on the ground, I see the wall, etc.); *proprioception*, where is my body in space (e.g., without looking, I sense my hand moving to touch my nose); and *interoception*, how do I feel internally (I feel hungry/tired/vibration/breath/other internal sensations). Voice work is highly internally focused. Teachers frequently ask, "How does this feel? What are your sensations?" Cultivating interoception is a critical component for sound-building; yet, for singers living in constant hyperarousal or freeze states, paying constant attention to internal sensation may become difficult, obsessive, or dissociative. Individuals that have experienced trauma may be over-, or under-stimulated by their internal sensations, unable to come back to the surface of the body and hold onto what is happening in the moment. For singers who express difficulty connecting outside experience (exteroception) with internal sensation (vibration, breath, heartbeat, emotion), providing a scaffolding for anchoring the body-mind in the present moment can be an invaluable resource. It can be a tremendous act of bravery to notice how breath and sound move in the body.

The process of dual awareness (or pendulation)—shifting our consciousness back and forth between two perceptions—can help us to access internal sensation while staying grounded more easily in the here and now. I feel my feet on the floor, as well as my breath; I can focus on a fixed point outside of my body while also sensing into vibration in my torso; I feel my breath moving internally while maintaining awareness of my hands at my side. These examples of dual awareness can allow us to explore internal sensations without becoming untethered. Over time, we may be able to sit with more uncomfortable sensations because we know that we have a container on the outside of our bodies to hold emotional and physical intensity.

Straw phonation is a wonderful example of incorporating dual awareness into voice practice. We can slowly pivot between what we experience externally (straw, bubbles, holding a glass) and internally (a steady flow of air and sound). If an internal sensation becomes too stimulating, we can always return to the exterior of the body and ground ourselves in the present moment. With patience and practice, singers can explore the relationship between bubbles and small sensations on their lips. This might slowly expand to observing both bubbles and feeling vibration around the face, as well as movement in the torso during exhalation. By titrating external awareness (water) with small internal cues (subtle airflow, movement, and buzzing), singers experiencing overwhelm can widen their capacity to experience interoceptive vocal sensations with less numbness or hypervigilance—and a bit of joy, as blowing bubbles can feel whimsical and child-like! Which of your favorite techniques could you adapt for mindfully exploring external and internal awareness? Intentional practice tools, along with the language that we use to describe technique, sensation, and application, invite an atmosphere of co-harmony. Trauma-informed voice care promotes vocal dignity by offering choices about *if*, *when*, and *how much* singers access sensation. Establishing boundaries around perception creates an external scaffolding for internal exploration.

Acknowledging how complex stress can manifest in the body, trauma-informed voice care provides an opportunity for voice professionals to examine how we hold space for our students. By noticing areas of disconnection and discomfort in our own bodies, we can make considered choices about how our words and practices invite well-being, continually affirming that all bodies, all voices, deserve to take up physical and acoustic space. The vital work of co-harmonization encourages us to be fully in the moment, welcoming any sensation that arises, and cultivating an environment of reciprocal trust, presence, and creativity. We are always guests in our students' physical, energetic, and acoustic spaces. Our visiting role is not to correct, fix, or answer, but to observe, offer, and empower. There is no technique more transformational than offering students the gift of a co-harmonizing supportive presence. In this way, our essential function shifts from I am here to teach to *I am here*.

An Overview of the Trauma-Informed Speech Pathologist
Carol Krusemark, CCC-SLP, PAVA-RV
Massachusetts General Hospital

I am a voice-specialized speech/language pathologist in a voice-dedicated clinic in Boston, Massachusetts. I have spent the past fourteen years working exclusively with clients needing voice rehabilitation. My client caseload has included vocalists, actors, teachers, attorneys, clergy members, employees of call centers, and other vocally demanding professions. It is a job I love, blending my love of singing with my chosen field of speech/language pathology.

While issues of voice and mental health have always coincided in my client census, over the past ten years, I began to notice that my clients, particularly young vocal performers, were increasingly anxious and depressed. I saw the same pattern in the graduate-level student clinicians that fulfilled a practicum at our facility. At the same time, I noticed that the voice-related tools I had at my disposal were not consistently working for these clients. Having come up in the field of speech/language pathology when it was pretty disorder-centric and tools and strategies focused, I felt at a loss. I had neither the insight nor the tools to help. Something seemed to interfere with the voice-specific tools I knew worked with others. I was frustrated. I began to question my worth as a voice therapist and, worse, blamed my clients for their lack of success.

Around this time, I realized how emotional trauma could impact a person's worldview, cognition, learning, self-concept, and ability to regulate. The ramifications for voice therapy seemed clear. Once I realized this, I began to recognize that many of my clients were coming to treatment in an activated state: a state in which they could neither self-assess, process sound or sensation, nor follow a suggested prompt. No wonder the "tools weren't working."

I began a deep dive into the concept of trauma-informed care before I understood what the term meant [*the principles of trauma-informed care appear in their entirety in chapter 6*]. As I continued to learn, trauma-informed care concepts seemed crucial to add to my work with clients and across the broader field of speech pathology and other healthcare professions. Adopting the principles of trauma-informed care has revolutionized my voice therapy practice. My clients are more engaged in their therapy process, clearer on their goals, and achieve their goals more quickly. I also find more job satisfaction and experience far less frustration and burnout. Instead of "taking my work home" with me in a way that negatively impacts my personal life, I feel energized, and my home-life balance has improved.

I believe the principles of trauma-informed care should be considered a "universal precaution" in healthcare. Just like washing hands and wearing gloves maximizes patient and provider safety, trauma-informed care principles provide a "way of being" with clients that maximizes safety and treatment success.

The term *trauma* currently means many things to many people. For this reason, I choose to use the definition of trauma provided by the Substance Abuse and Mental Health Services Administration (SAMHSA), which is worth directly quoting: "Individual trauma results from an event, series of events, or set of circumstances that is experienced by an individual as physically or emotionally harmful or life-threatening and that has lasting adverse effects on the individual's functioning and mental, physical, social, emotional, or spiritual well-being." Events, series of events, and sets of circumstances that *could* be experienced as physically or emotionally harmful or life-threatening occur at an astonishingly high rate in our larger culture. More than half of adults polled identified at least one potentially traumatic "adverse childhood event," and fully 25 percent described at least two ACEs, as they've come to be known. This does not take into account potentially trauma-inducing events that occur in adulthood. While not every individual exposed to adverse events develops emotional trauma, can we assume that everyone sitting in the chair opposite us has not been somehow impacted by challenging life events? Are we really only treating that "other" 50 percent?

Four of the overarching understandings outlined by SAMHSA now form the backbone of my client interactions: a realization of the prevalence of trauma, recognition of the signs and symptoms of trauma, response utilizing a trauma-informed approach to care, and avoidance of re-traumatization. Distinct from trauma-specific services or treatment, the principles of trauma-informed care comprise a "way of being" with and for our clients. The integral principles of a trauma-informed care approach that I have found most impactful to date include [the following]:

1. Creation of physical, mental, and psychological safety
2. Being true to my word and consistent with policies, and communication
3. Adopting a collaborative model of treatment, leveling the traditional clinician/client power differential
4. Taking the lead from my client and using a strengths-based approach to treatment as much as is possible
5. Understanding my multiple privileges, which helps me better hear and respect each client's lived experience with a voice problem and with the healthcare system in which I work. We are in a critical period in the allied health and more expansive medical health fields, where it will be increasingly important to move from a disorder-centric to a human-centric healthcare model. The policies, procedures, and practices of trauma-informed care are relevant aspects of universal design to adopt as we strive to meet the challenge of transforming our clinical relationships.

Notes

1. Deborah Caputo Rosen, Jonathan Brandon Sataloff, and Robert Thayer Sataloff, *Psychology of Voice Disorders*, second edition (San Diego: Plural Publishing. 2021), 223–24.
2. In her Movement for Trauma work, coach Jane Clapp suggests that the term "co-harmony" or "co-rhythm" may be a more suitable choice.
3. Stephen Porges, "Social Connectedness as a Biological Imperative" (handout from Butler University, September 21, 2019).
4. Staci Haines, *The Politics of Trauma* (Berkeley: North Atlantic Books, 2019), 74.
5. G. Berntson, J. T. Cacioppo, and K. S. Quigley, "Autonomic Determinism: The Modes of Autonomic Control, the Doctrine of Autonomic Space, and the Laws of Autonomic Constraint," *Psychology Review* 98, no. 4 (October 1991): 459–87.
6. Yana Hoffman, "Sing in the Shower to Make Friends with Your Vagus Nerve," *Psychology Today*, https://www.psychologytoday.com/us/blog/try-see-it-my-way/202003/sing-in-the-shower-make-friends-your-vagus-nerve. Accessed March 17, 2020.
7. Pat Ogden, *Trauma and the Body: A Sensorimotor Approach to Psychotherapy* (New York: W.W. Norton, 2006), 30–31.
8. Stephen Porges, "The Polyvagal Theory: New Insights into Adaptive Reactions of the Autonomic Nervous System," *Cleveland Clinic Journal of Medicine* 76, no. 2 (April 2009):86–S90.
9. Resmaa Menakem, *My Grandmother's Hands: Racialized Trauma and the Pathway to Mending Our Hearts and Bodies* (Las Vegas: Central Recovery Press, 2017), 14.
10. Peter Levine, *Waking the Tiger: Healing Trauma* (Berkeley: North Atlantic Books, 1997), 20.
11. "Concept of Trauma and Guidance for a Trauma Informed Approach," Substance Abuse and Mental Health Services Administration, https://ncsacw.samhsa.gov/userfiles/files/SAMHSA_Trauma.pdf. Accessed September 15, 2020.
12. "Mental Health by the Numbers," National Alliance on Mental Illness, https://www.nami.org/mhstats. Accessed September 15, 2020.
13. Leah B. Helou, Clark Rosen, Wei Wang, and Katherine Verdolini Abbott, "Intrinsic Laryngeal Muscle Response to a Public Speech Preparation Stressor," *The Laryngoscope* 123, no. 11 (November 2013): 1525–43.
14. Rosen et al., *Psychology of Voice Disorders*, 223–24.
15. Dave Phillips, "The Military Wants Better Tests for PTSD. Speech Analysis Could Be the Answer," *New York Times Magazine*, April 22, 2019, https://www.nytimes.com/2019/04/22/magazine/veterans-ptsd-speech-analysis.html.
16. Sonya Renee Taylor, *The Body Is Not an Apology: The Power of Radical Self-Love* (Oakland: Berrett-Koehler, 2018), 40.
17. Glenn White, "The Science of Breath Retraining," Buteyko Breathing Clinics, https://www.buteyko breathing.nz/Principles-of-Breathing-Retraining.html. Accessed September 15, 2020.

18. K. V. Naveen et al., "Yoga Breathing through a Particular Nostril Increases Spatial Memory Scores without Lateralized Effects," *Psychological Reports* 81, no. 2 (October 1997): 555–61.

19. Huang, "Concept of Trauma and Guidance for a Trauma Informed Approach."

20. Ibid.

21. Ibid.

22. Ibid.

23. Betty Martin, "What Are We Doing?," https://bettymartin.org/?sermon=introduction. Last modified, July 27, 2022.

24. Travis Sherwood, "Inspiring Autonomous Artists: A Framework for Independent Singing," *Journal of Singing* 75, no. 5 (May/June 2019): 527.

25. Iris Yob, Estelle R. Jorgensen (eds.), *Humane Music Education for the Common Good* (Bloomington: Indiana University Press, 2020), 160–61.

26. Erich Fromm, *To Have or To Be* (New York: Harper & Row, 1976).

27. Deb Dana, *The Polyvagal Theory in Therapy: Engaging the Rhythm of Regulation* (New York: W. W. Norton, 2014), 44.

28. Jane Clapp, "Movement for Trauma Level One Training Manual" (syllabus, Toronto, ON, 2020), 20.

6

Ethical Scope of Practice

Emily Jaworski Koriath

> *More than anything else, being able to feel safe with other people defines mental health; safe connections are fundamental to meaningful and satisfying lives.*
>
> —Bessel van der Kolk[1]

[Disclosure: this chapter is authored by a voice teacher with a terminal degree in the field, who has also completed the multi-year training process to become a Somatic Experiencing (™) practitioner. While I do indeed see private clients for the express purpose of negotiating trauma, I *do not* practice trauma healing on the students I teach through my institution.]

AS A VOICE PROFESSIONAL, it is essential to remember that you're not a therapist, even though you may possess extraordinary empathy and excellent listening skills. As discussed in chapter 5, your job as a trauma-informed practitioner is not to heal trauma. Your job is to be aware of the prevalence of trauma and the ways that it can impact learning, relationships, and singing skills. Recall from chapter 3 that our most effective tool for healing is co-regulation, offering a stable nervous system for your students to be influenced by. As defined by the Center for Health Care Strategies,

Trauma-informed care seeks to:

- Realize the widespread impact of trauma and understand paths for recovery

- Recognize the signs and symptoms of trauma in patients, families, and staff
- Integrate knowledge about trauma into policies, procedures, and practices; and
- Actively avoid re-traumatization.[2]

The potential for re-traumatization in the voice studio is extremely high, especially if teachers reach beyond their scope and ask singers to recount their experiences in detail in a misguided attempt to "help" or to "heal." As described in chapter 1, reliving traumatic events activates the amygdala and the release of stress hormones, while also knocking out critical brain areas, making it highly likely that being asked about a traumatic experience will only cause a singer to relive it rather than providing any therapeutic value.[3]

Van der Kolk described a study conducted in the early 1990s with veterans suffering from PTSD (posttraumatic stress disorder). One element of the study required the participants to speak repeatedly about every detail of their experiences in Vietnam. Patients became panicked by flashbacks and reported depression and dread lasting for many days after each session. The study was brought to a halt because so many patients dropped out and never returned. Many of the volunteers who stayed with the study became increasingly violent and fearful.[4] Van der Kolk explains: "I've learned that it's not important for me to know every detail of a patient's trauma. What is critical is that the patients themselves learn to tolerate feeling what they feel and knowing what they know."[5] I put it to readers that if a trained doctor with over forty years of experience in the field of trauma studies doesn't need to know the details of a client's history in order to provide meaningful support, then we as voice teachers don't either.

Van der Kolk goes on to explain that becoming a competent trauma therapist requires learning about the impact of trauma, abuse, and neglect, and developing a variety of techniques that can help to "(1) stabilize and calm patients down, (2) help to lay traumatic memories and reenactments to rest, and (3) reconnect patients with their fellow [humans]."[6] Therapists also embark on their own process of intensive therapy, as a mandatory part of their training. This work enables therapists to maintain a sense of empathy with patients while also holding clients' experiences at a safe distance. While voice teachers spend intense one-on-one time with singers in the studio, and while we sometimes hold space for students to vent difficult emotions or tell the truth about the stories they carry, we are not adequately trained to heal their trauma.

Of Special Note: Transference and Countertransference
From Elisa Monti, Ph.D.

When interacting with others, sometimes we deal with factors that operate below our consciousness. The exchanges we have with other individuals can be influenced by the psychological history of the person we are interacting with (whether a peer, a student, or anyone) and by our own history. The influencing factors coming from the student or peer can be referred to as "transference," and the forces entered into the space by us in response are our "countertransference." These terms may ring a bell for the reader but are generally only taught and utilized when it comes to psychotherapy. In reality these phenomena can take place in any interaction.

"Transference" refers to associations in which past dynamics are reflected into current relationships.[1] For example, a student in a singing lesson might feel the need to justify and over-explain any "mistake" that occurs during the lesson. This might happen, for example, if that was something this individual had to do growing up when interacting with the adults around them. The image and feelings evoked by those adults become "transferred" onto the voice teacher. The voice teacher, in turn, might feel compelled to reassure the student constantly and make the interaction appear as safe as possible at every turn. This could certainly be influenced by simple compassion; but if other layers exist to this need to reassure and keep the student safe—for example if the voice teacher had to do this with siblings when very young—this would then be the teacher's "countertransference." This is the term "used when therapists respond to the patients' transference issues with transference issues of their own."[2] These dynamics can occur in all interactions, not just psychotherapeutic.[3] Certainly, we cannot claim that all reactions are informed by transference or countertransference elements. However, it is imperative to reflect on the (often layered) origin of elements we introduce in dynamics.

Sometimes, the result can be mixed.[4] Ultimately, reflecting on these factors can help us help the person we are working with.[5] Psychotherapists often use such factors as part of their analysis of a client. Indeed, a voice teacher will use this awareness very differently, just as they do with the student's trauma history. Nonetheless, only by maintaining the awareness that deeper layers might be at play in any exchange, the teacher will stay with the totality of the human experience when teaching.

Notes

1. Alun C. Jones, "Transference and Countertransference," Perspectives on Psychiatric Care, 40, no.1 (January 2004) 13–19.
2. Ibid., 14.
3. Ibid.
4. Austin, Diane. The theory and practice of vocal psychotherapy: Songs of the self. Jessica Kingsley Publishers, 2009.
5. Ibid.

For years mumbles have been heard throughout the voice teacher community about the fact that "anyone can hang out a shingle" and call themselves a voice teacher. This creates numerous challenges for the profession, especially when singers report vocal damage or emotional abuse while engaged in voice work with a particular teacher. The closest thing we have to a governing body is the National Association of Teachers of Singing (NATS), the largest professional organization of singing teachers in the world, with over seven thousand members in thirty-seven countries. There are several other noteworthy organizations contributing to the advancement of the profession, such as the American Academy of Teachers of Singing, the New York Singing Teachers' Association, and the Pan-American Vocology Association, among many others. NATS has done well creating a code of ethics for its members (the most recent edition was approved in 2018), but it is important to remember that not every voice professional is a member of NATS. The difficulties this presents, and the no doubt countless discussions that have taken place around tables and meeting rooms for decades, are well beyond the scope of this text. However, there is some critical history from the last decade that is worth summarizing to illustrate how we've arrived at this moment in voice care.

Joint Statement from NATS, ASHA, and VASTA

In 2005, NATS, The American Speech-Language-Hearing Association (ASHA), and the Voice and Speech Trainers Association (VASTA) issued a joint statement on scope of practice titled "The Role of the Speech-Language Pathologist, the Teacher of Singing, and the Speaking Voice Trainer in Voice Habilitation."[7] That document began with acknowledging that historically, roles in voice care had been more siloed in practice, with (in the simplest of terms) recovery from laryngeal disorders being the purview of the SLP (speech-language pathologist), restoration of singing function the role of the teacher, and development of normal voices to maximum potential for use in performance or public speaking the domain of a speech trainer. However, the document went on to acknowledge that there was a growing consensus that this "separatist approach" might not be in the best interest of singers and speakers, and all three organizations affirmed "that the most effective path to vocal recovery often will include an integrated approach to optimal voice care and production that addresses both speech and singing tasks."

The statement went on to acknowledge that there are some speech pathologists who are experienced singers or teachers of singing, and some otolaryngologists are also members of ASHA, but such multiple specializations are rare and professional preparation varies greatly among these three areas of professional practice. The statement went on to advocate for the following adaptations (briefly summarized):

1. The preparation of the SLPs needs to be augmented to include instruction in vocal performance and vocal pedagogy to help clients "to develop both the singing voice and speaking voice to optimum levels of health, performance, and artistry."
2. The preparation of the teachers of singing needs to be augmented in a comparable manner to include training in anatomy and physiology, behavioral management of voice problems, development of the speaking voice, and the singing teacher's role in working with the speech-language pathologist and the physician in the medical management of voice disorders.
3. Similarly, the preparation of voice and speech trainers who work with singers and other professional speakers needs to include instruction in anatomy and physiology, behavioral management of voice problems, singing pedagogy and performance, and the voice and speech trainer's role in working with the speech-language pathologist and the physician in the medical management of voice disorders.

Perhaps most germane to the focus of this chapter, the statement ends with a crucial caveat, quoted in its entirety here (emphasis by the editor):

> ASHA, NATS, and VASTA recognize the existence of *state licensure laws* that govern delivery of services to persons with communication disorders, including voice disorders. *All persons* who work with speakers and singers with voice disorders are encouraged to become familiar with these laws. ASHA, NATS, and VASTA affirm that it remains the responsibility of the individual practitioner to ensure that his or her work with singers and other professional voice users does not violate the scope of practice defined by the laws in the state(s) where the work is done.

As of this writing, the lines between these professions have become even more blurred as teachers of singing become more scientifically informed, but this increase in training has perhaps led to more practitioners overstepping their individual scope. For example, though I have attended several lectures on vocal pathology, it would be completely inappropriate for me to say to a student "I think you have nodes," or "it sounds like you might have an injury so let's see what we can figure out." Only a laryngeal examination can conclusively determine the cause of a vocal issue. It is never a voice teacher's job to "guess" what's wrong based on what they covered in their vocal pedagogy course in graduate school.

Survey of Teachers

In 2006, speech pathologists Amy Fields and Edie Hapner (now my colleague at the University of Alabama at Birmingham) conducted a survey of SLPs who also treat singers. While there was little consensus among respondents about the qualifications necessary to treat singers, 89 percent of the fifty-seven speech-language pathologists who reported treating voice disorders in singers had completed additional degrees in music and/or had at least two years of private vocal training, and only 10 percent reported no performing experience and little (less than one year) or no vocal training.[8]

In 2010 Hapner teamed up with colleagues Marina Gilman and John Nix to conduct a similar survey of teachers of singing. That survey concluded that singing teachers collectively lacked specialized training in anatomy, physiology, and voice disorders and their effects on the singing voice. The writers also noted that there is "no single professional group with expertise in anatomy and physiology of laryngeal structure and function, voice disorders and their impact on laryngeal structure and function, and habilitation and/rehabilitation of the singing voice." In the simplest of terms, *habilitation* refers to the enhancement of a healthy, functioning voice, and *rehabilitation* refers to the restoration of function in a disordered voice. The writers also acknowledged that while the Voice Foundation has been working since the 1970s to unite the medical, SLP, and voice teacher communities to enhance the collaborative treatment of singers with vocal pathology,

> there remains little agreement on the skills and credentials needed to treat singers with voice pathologies after diagnosis and medical treatment by the otolaryngologist. While the American Speech-Language and Hearing Association has developed the certificate of clinical competence, and while most states require licensure for speech-language pathologists to practice, there are not competencies, guidelines, or licensure for singing teachers.

Symposium at the National Center for Voice and Speech

In 2013, several groups of stakeholders including physicians, speech-language pathologists, voice teachers, choral conductors, speech and voice trainers, and performers met in Utah to discuss the potential for a proposed specialty training in vocal health.[9] The symposium had two major goals: (1) to clarify the titles used in the realm of vocal health reflect a provider's qualifications so that members of the public can more easily identify the types of professionals who can meet their needs, and (2) to improve the specificity of language used to describe the roles and responsibilities of voice care providers "so that the public is adequately informed of the provider's level of education, training, experience, depth of scientific and clinical knowledge, and scope of practice."

Symposium attendees discussed the popularity of the term "singing voice specialist," in heavy use at the time, and felt that this title did not denote an identity separate from that of a singing teacher. The term "vocologist," though not formally recognized in the medical world, could be used to more readily identify someone steeped in the principles of vocal habilitation through experience performing or teaching, as well as advanced knowledge of voice science; someone capable of both vocal habilitation and rehabilitation. The conversation then progressed to the potential for creating a vocologist credential, and possible vocologist training programs, which would include the following:

- anatomy of the upper body, and specifically the head and neck region
- an introduction to the biomechanics of tissue and air movement
- principles of sound production and propagation in airways (acoustics)
- physiology of breathing, vocalization, and natural sound reinforcement
- scientific concepts of motor learning and theories of practice as they might be applied to voice training and practice regimens
- training to hear small changes in the vocal signal, relating perception to production through personal performance experience, the use of visual cues (posture, alignment, strain, tension, freedom of movement)
- the use of instrumentation for voice analysis
- a thorough knowledge and understanding of voice disorders.
- understanding and being able to classify voice pathologies and voice limitations
- systemic effects of disease and medications on the voice, the difference between medical diagnoses and functional assessment, and a spectrum of therapy techniques (e.g., vocal exercises, laryngeal manipulation, and nutrition).

Symposium attendees noted that there were two potential pathways for undertaking the roles described as the work of a vocologist: SLPs with previous experience in performing or training of performing voices and singing teachers "who have sought out extra training in vocal health, voice science, and vocology."

Lastly, there followed an extensive discussion of the ethics and responsibilities of the emerging profession of vocology:

> Considerations include liability of the provider of vocal habilitation and rehabilitation, insurance billing and medical ethics, and regulation of practitioners. One of the invited speakers was an attorney who gave a presentation on liability and healthcare providers, and indicated that, at least under Utah law, anyone purporting to provide rehabilitation of injury is subject to malpractice liability.

It became clear that if the term vocologist was to become formalized, there needed to be an organization capable of defining the role of the vocologist and establishing standards for training. As a result, the Pan-American Vocology Association (PAVA) was created to "establish a codified set of standards, scope of practice, and eventually oversee certification."[10] In 2022, PAVA announced the creation of a process whereby individuals can earn the credential of PAVA-Recognized Vocologist, or PAVA-RV, and as of this writing, several vocology training programs have been created to provide this level of training. This careful delineation of roles and scope of practice is crucial as more voice professionals adopt the lens of trauma-informed care. It bears continued repeating that the aim of this text is not to create voice teachers who overstep their professional boundaries and attempt to heal any singer's trauma.

Professional Ethics

As we look to apply trauma-informed principles to voice work, it's valuable to consider the code of ethics of two closely related professional agencies: ASHA, and the American Psychological Association (APA). Both organizations have crafted a robust code of professional standards that will also serve the trauma-informed voice practitioner. We'll draw from these codes of ethics, as well as the most recent code of ethics from NATS, as a frame for adapting the six core principles of a trauma-informed approach introduced in chapter 5. They are as follows:[11]

1. Safety
2. Trustworthiness and transparency
3. Peer support
4. Collaboration and mutuality
5. Empowerment, voice, and choice
6. Cultural, historical, and gender issues

The NATS code of ethics consists of three sections: Personal Ethical Standards, Ethical Standards Relating to Students, and Ethical Standards Relating to Colleagues. Here are the two items most relevant to trauma-informed practice:

1. Members shall present themselves honestly, in a dignified and professional manner, and with documented qualifications. These may include appropriate academic degrees, awards, professional affiliations, and teaching and performing experience. And
2. Members should maintain appropriate boundaries in psychological, emotional, and personal contact with students, including insinuations that could be construed as sexual advances, even when a student may encourage or *request* such interaction.[12]

These two points serve as essential reminders to voice professionals that claiming to possess psychological training or involving oneself in psychological and emotional matters without clear boundaries is unethical. This does not mean that we must shut down our empathy, or silence students who need a safe place to voice frustrations or difficult experiences. As you'll recall from chapter 1, suppressing emotions leads to tension in the body, and tension in the body will almost certainly impact vocal production. It's not the voice teacher's job to solicit an emotional outpouring from students, but if a student happens to share that they are going through something difficult, a teacher can ethically and responsibly hear that information without involving oneself in problem solving or offering advice. In the 2021 publication *Teaching the Whole Musician: A Guide to Wellness in the Applied Studio*, author Paola Savvidou shares skills and tools based on her experiences leading the Wellness Initiative at the University of Michigan School of Music. While the entire book is a worthy addition to the field, perhaps most relevant to trauma-informed pedagogy is Savvidou's inclusion of motivational interviewing, a style of communication that involves empathic listening and helping a person discover their own intrinsic needs and wants.[13] While anyone can become trained in motivational interviewing, Savvidou beautifully adapts the principles (including sample scripts) for the applied studio. The approach she advocates in *Teaching the Whole Musician* encourages the teacher to listen deeply, and then to ask the student what they are hoping to gain from the conversation. Some students want advice or to hear strategies that other students have utilized when facing similar challenges. Others may just want to be heard. The principles of motivational interviewing provide an excellent framework for ethically engaging in emotional conversations with students.

There may also come a time where a student discloses something that is well beyond our scope of practice, like disordered eating or self-harming behaviors. If a student trusts you enough to share this information with you, it is important to honor this trust and your professional obligations simultaneously. I always begin by asking my students what support they already have in place. Some of them are engaged in a relationship with a helping professional like a social worker or a therapist and don't need interventions from me. Sometimes sharing this information is part of a very intentional healing process. Many teachers put up a wall around information like this because they are scared. We don't need to be scared; we need to honor our own boundaries and make them clear to students. Most of the time, what students are seeking by sharing their truth is someone who can listen and who can sit with them in the complexity of the situation. While a therapist or other helping professional will be working with the student on root causes and coping strategies, you can help them to strategize how to manage their work around their emotional lives. For example, how do their panic attacks impact their work? Which people in their life should be notified about a disorder like that, and how can they communicate their experience and their needs, so they feel less shame and stigma about their emotional world? Bravery and boundaries are required to be able to enter these types of conversations, because we don't know what will happen and we might not feel ready. But when we can sit with students and truly listen to what they are sharing and what they need, we provide essential co-regulation, compassion, and clear-headed presence that shows that we are not afraid of witnessing the messy parts of their worlds.

Lauren A. Cook provides a template based on her experience with disordered eating behaviors, but the basic outline can apply to numerous forms of student disclosure.

> If a student discloses that they have an eating disorder, there is no reason to suspend teaching or teach any differently until they recover unless it has been prescribed/suggested by a medical professional. Here are a few things to keep in mind:
>
> - Ask the student if they would like to continue lessons. Does singing help or harm? For some, singing is a release and necessary to recovery. For others, the singing and performing can be wrapped up in the psychology of the disorder. Try, as schedule and finances permit, to be flexible with them.
> - Have them see an otolaryngologist if they have not already. Purging disorders can wreak havoc on the digestive system, and just like GERD (gastroesophageal reflux disease) or LPR (laryngopharyngeal reflux), may affect laryngeal function. Restrictive disorders can result in severely decreased energy and strength, and may cause accessory muscles to overwork, causing overuse injuries.
> - Be mindful of where mirrors are in your studio and how often you ask students to stand in front of them. Can a shoulders-up or compact mirror get the same job done? Ask how they would feel about using a mirror for a certain concept. Accept that they might say no.
> - Try to avoid your own negative body talk or discussion of intentional weight loss in the studio. (This is a good guideline to always follow, but particularly with this population.) Do not offer suggestions regarding diet or exercise.
>   - If you have personal experience with disordered eating, you do not need to feel obligated to disclose this to your student. This will greatly depend on where you are in your recovery and your relationship with the student.
>   - If you feel this student may indirectly affect your own recovery, you may want to refer them to another teacher for the time being.
> - Do your best to avoid complimenting appearance and/or weight changes.

- Do not offer recovery-based incentives (e.g., "If you follow your meal plan you can sing in the recital!").
- Know that recovery is a long process and not a linear process. Your student will have good days and bad days, and just as you would for any other student, hold space for them. You are under no obligation to discuss the topic with the student but needn't avoid it if the student brings it up. Use any strategies you normally would for students who tend to overshare or under share.
- More resources can be found at the National Eating Disorder Association (NEDA), https://www.nationaleatingdisorders.org/. They also have an excellent hotline and can answer questions and provide professional support.

What to Do If You Suspect a Student Has an Eating Disorder

- If the student is a minor, a separate phone call or discussion with the parent/caregiver *outside of the lesson time* and first without the student present can be helpful. It's possible the parents know, but it's also possible they are in denial or unaware. Do not diagnose, but share your concerns for the student's overall health, vocal health, and well-being.
- If the student is in college or another academic program, it's usually best to first talk to your department chair. There may already be protocol in place for students who are suffering with mental or physical illness. This will possibly then go to their residence director or student affairs, depending on the university's policies. If you and your department chair feel it is appropriate for you to bring this directly to the student's attention, do it outside of lesson time. Taking up lesson time can send the message that the outcome of the discussion or next steps may change the professional working relationship. I would not have this discussion without informing your supervisor/department chair/coordinator first.
- If it is a private student over the age of eighteen, you may have to decide where your professional boundaries are. There is no right or wrong answer. If you feel it is appropriate to have a conversation, using the NEDA resources can be very helpful. If you feel it is out of your scope of practice, that is also okay. It will often depend on your relationship with the student and there is not a one-size-fits-all approach.

As we consider motivational interviewing and other techniques of value, it is worth noting that our colleagues in ASHA are ethically bound to continue developing high-level skills to serve their clients:

D. Individuals shall enhance and refine their professional competence and expertise through engagement in lifelong learning applicable to their professional activities and skills.[14]

While a set of core competencies for vocal educators may never be argued into existence, I might offer some suggestions about elements of vocal work that feel essential for all students.

Fundamentals of Human Breathing

Teachers must understand how breathing actually works in human bodies. Where does air go when we breathe in? And how does that air leave the body as sound? Another reason to update your understanding of breathing is that "[s]cientific methods have confirmed that changing the way one breathes can improve problems with anger, depression, and anxiety,"[15] but only when that breathing is based on credible science. Breathing "from the diaphragm" is physically impossible and clenching the butt cheeks is not sustainable vocal technique. (Recommended resources include Jessica Wolf's "Art of Breathing" website; *The Humanual* and *The Actor's Secret* by Betsy Polatin; and *Breath: The New Science of a Lost Art* by James Nestor.)

Enough Anatomical Truth to Teach Alignment in Cooperation with Human Design

Telling students to pull their shoulders back creates tension across the muscles of the chest and restricts breathing. Asking students to lift their heads toward the ceiling as if pulled by string causes constriction in the muscles of the neck and compromises the vocal tract. When some people are given the cue to "ground," they simply initiate a downward collapse of the entire upper body. (Recommended resources include investing in some Alexander Technique lessons, especially those taught by AT teachers with singing experience; and exploring Body Mapping with a licensed teacher.)

Style Parameters for a Variety of Applications

Gone are the days when singing training = classical technique only. Though this certainly was not true even twenty years ago, thanks to pioneers like Jeannette LoVetri and others, there is now a host of evidence-based pedagogical tools for musical theater, jazz, gospel, pop, and even rock screaming. (Recommended resources include LoVetri, who offers her own series of workshops in Somatic Voicework(R), and the CCM Institute at Shenandoah University, which offers both a multi-level curriculum in CCM pedagogy and continuing education courses every summer. If your classical technique hasn't been refreshed in a while, there's a summer institute at Westminster Choir College. W. Stephen Smith wrote a fantastic book called *The Naked Voice: A Wholistic Approach to Singing*, and professional development programs are available through NYSTA, NYU's online school of continuing ed, and PAVA and NATS continually offer webinars for educators. In the summer of 2023, NATS ran their first sponsored Science-Informed Pedagogy Institute, and noted pedagogue Ian Howell offers professional development programs through the new Embodied Music Lab. NATS has also published an extensive collection of scinece-informed pedagogy resources, available at https://www.nats.org/cgi/page.cgi/Science-Informed_Voice_Pedagogy_Resources.html. But of critical importance is that we incorporate this scientific understanding in cooperation with our emphasis on expressive skills; if you only focus on the properties of sound production, your students are only learning a small part of the job of a skilled performer.

Professional Ethics and the Principles of Trauma-Informed Practice

Following is an in-depth discussion of the core principles of a trauma-informed approach to care, adapted from the Substance Abuse and Mental Health Services Administration's "Trauma-Informed Approach."[16] These principles have also been endorsed by the U.S. Centers for Disease Control (CDC), and at present no fewer than thirty government agencies are collaborating as the Interagency Task Force for Trauma-Informed Care,[17] charged with gathering data and recommending best practices.

1. Safety

Some thoughts on safety from the APA Code of Ethics:

3.04 Avoiding Harm[18]
(a) Psychologists take reasonable steps to avoid harming their clients/patients, students, supervisees, research participants, organizational clients, and others with whom they work, and to minimize harm where it is foreseeable and unavoidable.

> *Someone who is stern, judgmental, agitated, or harsh is likely to leave you feeling scared, abandoned, and humiliated, and that won't help you resolve your traumatic stress.*
>
> —Bessel van der Kolk[19]

Verbally abusing students with the aim of "toughening them up" is harmful. Telling students that they will never succeed is harmful. Telling students in fat bodies that they are unacceptable is harmful. True, the performing arts industry can be cruel and at the worst of times, abusive. But as we will repeat throughout this text, resilience skills come *after* safety and stability are established. While it is negligent not to let students know about the potential difficulties they may face as they emerge into the professional landscape, there is no reason for you to treat them abusively "for their own good."

There are several concepts that we can put into practice in the studio to create what is known in school research as a "climate of care." As Stanford senior lecturer and education researcher Denise Pope wrote in *Overloaded and Underprepared*,

> At a time when national estimates suggest that 20 to 25 percent of adolescents are experiencing symptoms of emotional distress, including depression, anxiety, self-mutilation, and substance abuse, the need to identify school and classroom-based practices that adolescents perceive as supportive and caring has become a matter of great urgency and importance.[20]

While Pope's research focuses on public schools, it applies to undergraduate populations as well. Until every high school environment evolves to meet students' emotional needs, university teachers need to take up the charge. This climate of care is imperative based on what we, as teachers of emerging artists, know about our students and the emotional challenges they face. If we can't allow singers to fully be themselves, we can't possibly expect that they will be able to dig deep into human emotion to find something compelling to convey about a piece. Pope goes on to remind educators that learning depends on a student's "physical state, personal comfort, emotional health, mindset, and preferred learning style," and therefore it's crucial that students feel safe and cared for in school, that they have supportive mentors who encourage them to take risks and learn from mistakes, and that they learn about wellness and stress management.[21]

Teachers must conduct a fearless assessment of the actual safety of their studio. It does little to hang a "Safe Space" sticker on your door if you are not willing to listen empathetically to students and hear their needs without judgment. Could you hold space for a student who is experiencing difficulties? Can you hear what students are saying without focusing on your own discomfort first? This is admittedly difficult work, but as we discussed in chapter 2, our students (and their nervous systems) know the difference between people who proclaim to be safe and those who actually are. The type of environment we need to strive to create and protect is one of *psychological safety*. This term was first coined by Harvard organizational and behavioral scientist Amy Edmondson, who defines psychologically safe environments as those places where one can show oneself without fear of consequences to their self-image or career, and where the climate is characterized by trust and mutual respect. Psychological safety does not mean that we stop telling our students the truth. It means that teachers hold the understanding that some truths are difficult to hear, and some students may react negatively to criticism. This doesn't mean that we give up on these difficult conversations. It means that we engage in tough talks with compassion and empathy. We tell the truth and offer follow-up plans or emotional support based on what the student needs most at that moment. We can't shield students from the truth, but we also can't ignore that some truths are painful and take time to digest. [22]

We need to be able to provide this kind of atmosphere for students because in most cases, their creativity has not been nurtured or encouraged in school, especially in light of the enormous disruptions to learning caused by the COVID-19 pandemic. Every singer has their own unique brand of creativity, and with the right tools, every teacher can teach students how to build on those gifts. Teachers also need to cultivate their *own* creativity so that they can be intuitive and flexible in lessons. We have to honor how people actually are, and this means that they will sometimes surprise us, and we need to create an environment of freedom, flexibility, and ease.

2. Trustworthiness and Transparency

Create a Culture of Exploration and Discovery

After my first faculty recital at UAB, a student was stunned to learn that things were still hard for me to learn and prepare. I told them that having a doctorate didn't mean that I had everything figured out. Just like any singer, I have my unique old habits and curious little hang ups. The biggest difference is that now I know how to look out for those things, and when they arise, I have a finely honed set of tools I can employ to get more of what I want in my singing. I took out my binder and showed them the copious markings and notes to myself that covered my scores: shorthand markings I've developed, symbols I use, and sometimes, narrative prose about what or how to practice. In *The Teacher's Ego*, Eustis writes that if students know that you as the teacher are experimenting and trying to find the ideal approach to the challenges presented in the repertoire, they will be more likely to adopt this mindset in their own practicing and exploration.[23] Julia Cameron, author of *The Artist's Way* and numerous other titles on creativity, hints at the freedom and joy that can come from this type of reframing: "When we focus on ourselves as works in progress, we regain a sense of adventure and fulfillment. We embrace change as integral to our continual process of unfolding."[24]

Lynn Eustis modeled this for me. I find her to be an impeccably prepared singer at all times. She sings accurately but always musically, and with a gorgeous tone employed by an elegant hand. She still performs often and was always generous about sharing the challenges of a particular piece, or new observations gleaned through the work. To me, this was the embodiment of something she said often in the studio: she's not in the teacher's chair because she has all the answers, she's just been walking down the road longer.

I've brought this approach into my studio as well. Like many teachers I know, I've gained numerous practical tools after being disappointed and frustrated by my voice for many years. I've learned a lot by refusing to accept that my voice couldn't do what I wanted it to, and it's just my nature that when I learn things, I want to tell people about them. I want them to have an easier time than I did, so they can make choices about what they are learning sooner than I did. Like many developing singers whose voices don't easily fit into established categories, I got two degrees and did roles, auditions, and competitions *singing the wrong voice part.* I did the best I could with the information I had, but I still sometimes wonder what could or would have happened if I had gained some answers sooner. I can't change the past, and with time, that confusion and hurt has faded. It still appears acutely here and there when a good friend or colleague has a big success that I read about on social media, but I wasn't equipped for a big career when I was younger. I had no idea what I didn't know and how much more there was to learn about my voice. Now that I know more, I sing what I want, and I sing as much as I want. There is a part of me that thinks that even if I had built a different kind of performing career, I would have ended up in this same place: doing what I want and trying to help others do the same.

I've begun using the word "exploration" in a very deliberate way in the studio. If a student comes in with questions about a particular concept, I say, "Let's try a little bit of exploration and see what we can figure out." I frame us as co-conspirators: we're in it together, flipping over rocks, poking things with sticks, and bouncing ideas off each other to see what works. As Cameron teaches in *The Artist's Way at Work*, "increased creativity is a teachable, trackable process. . . . All of us can become more creative than we already are, and this will make us happier, healthier, more productive, and more authentic in everything we do."[25] We never really know what will happen. What Dr. Eustis showed me in our four years together is that I was there to do the work—and to be changed. On several occasions (every week?), when I told her that I needed to quit the program, she encouraged me to stay the course, so that when I was finished, I would have my degree *and then I could do whatever I want.* That part was a new concept to me. The doctorate didn't set the path; *I* got a degree on my path, and then I could just keep going.

Perhaps the first musician to write about creativity in the learning process was Eloise Ristad, a piano teacher whose groundbreaking book *A Soprano on*

Her Head was written almost forty years ago. I can't remember who recommended it to me in that very nebulous time after I completed my master's degree, but it was the first time I had read anything about music that suggested that I might have ideas and that those ideas might actually be useful in music making. Ristad wrote that it may seem easier (especially at the end of a long teaching day, or week, or semester) to just give students answers, but what happens then is that we rob them of the opportunity to try and fail and try again, ultimately arriving at something wholly their own that they can recall and apply to future problems. "If the student is part of the process of discovery . . . the solution to a problem then becomes a personal triumph."[26] Certainly, in terms of technique, there might be things I am inclined to suggest, but more and more I find myself pointing a neon arrow and asking things like "What do you know that could help you make a plan for that high note?" Then the student gets to draw on their experience in the studio or with other pieces and devise a strategy for problem solving. I remind them that I'll be there to help them evaluate that plan, and to help if they get stuck, but overall, I give them a good map, teach them to drive, and then point.

3. Peer Support

Disclosure of our own trauma histories is not required of us as voice professionals. If a student is experiencing difficulties, you can point to the importance of finding someone who has been through a similar experience. In *Anchored: Befriending Your Nervous System Using Polyvagal Theory*, Deb Dana offers teachers another frame through which we can view this principle. As teachers, we can provide context, choice, and connection which help the nervous system to find a sense of safety and balance. Dana points out that "[w]hen these three elements are present, we more easily find the way to regulation. When any one of these elements is missing, we feel off balance and experience a sense of unease." Dana explains:

> Through the lens of the nervous system, *context* involves gathering information about how, what, and why in order to understand, and respond to, experiences. . . . Without explicitly stated information, we are more likely to sense unsafety and move into a pattern of protection.
>
> With *choice*, it's possible to be still or move, approach or avoid, connect or protect. When choice is limited or taken away, or when we have a sense of being stuck or trapped without options, we begin to look for a way out.
>
> With *connection* we feel safely embodied, accompanied by others, at home in the environment, and in harmony with spirit. When there is a rupture in our sense of connection . . . our ability to anchor in safety and regulation is challenged, and we turn to communication and social engagement to try to find our way back into connection."[27]

As we'll discuss in chapter 8, when we revisit secure attachment, by practicing healthy connection in the studio, we help make future social connections easier. Van der Kolk underscores the necessity of social support by citing "numerous studies of disaster response around the globe have shown that social support is the most powerful protection against becoming overwhelmed by stress and trauma."[28] But he goes on to clarify that social support is not the same as simply being surrounded by others. You'll recall from chapter 3 that what humans really seek is a deep sense of being seen. Van der Kolk says, "The critical issue is *reciprocity*: being truly heard and seen by the people around us."[29]

4. Collaboration and Mutuality

From the APA:

> 7.04 Student Disclosure of Personal Information[30]
> Psychologists do not require students or supervisees to disclose personal information in course- or program-related activities, either orally or in writing, regarding sexual history, history of abuse and neglect, psychological treatment, and relationships with parents, peers, and spouses or significant others except if . . . the information is necessary to evaluate or obtain assistance for students whose personal problems could reasonably be judged to be preventing them from performing their training- or professionally related activities in a competent manner or posing a threat to the students or others.

Each institution has its own parameters on safe reporting, and what sorts of disclosure require an employee to report their concerns to others. Check your university's policies and consider writing your own if you are an independent studio teacher. However, as we'll discuss in this book's conclusion, there is a very real amount of harm that can be posed by institutions in response to student welfare. I worked with a student who was very aware of their mental health challenges and was working with a team of individuals to support them. They learned quickly that disclosing feelings of self-harming behaviors or suicidal ideation was a crucial component of being able to resist these impulses and remain safe. However, there was a very difficult period of learning exactly who were their most helpful allies in this process. On several occasions, this student notified an RA (resident assistant, usually a student who lives in a residence hall), and because this person was unaware of the student's history, they called the police according to their training. While the RA did not do anything wrong in this situation, my student was further traumatized by police officers without appropriate training to negotiate such crises; they were taken to a hospital emergency room and left alone for several hours while other more critical cases were tended to, according to standard emergency room procedures. Over time, this student developed a safe network of helping professionals, supportive peers, and internal tools to help them navigate this difficult period.

The Role of the Teacher in Emotional Skill Building

> *Since emotional regulation is the critical issue in managing the effects of trauma and neglect, it would make an enormous difference if teachers, army sergeants, foster parents, and mental health professionals were thoroughly schooled in emotional regulation techniques.*
>
> —Bessel van der Kolk[31]

Before any teacher embarks on the journey of folding emotional intelligence skills into the curriculum, we must take time to recall that there is an inherent power differential in the student-teacher relationship. Our students come to us to learn how to become artists, and emotional skills are an essential professional skill. We are not therapists, and under no circumstances should we require students to be emotionally vulnerable *for no reason*. We also cannot use their questions and their struggles against them when we get frustrated. Difficult as it may be, we must also refrain from offering unsolicited advice on students' relationships or mental health. Remember that the most effective support teachers can offer is powerful, steady co-regulation; being present to all the thoughts and feelings that arise in our students without judgment, assessment, or the impulse to "fix." We return to bell hooks for powerful guidance on the delicate nature of this balance:

> Any classroom that employs a holistic model of learning will also be a place where teachers grow, and are empowered by the process. That empowerment cannot happen if we refuse to be vulnerable while encouraging students to take risks. Professors who expect students to share confessional narratives but who are themselves unwilling to share are exercising power in a manner that could be coercive. . . . When professors bring narratives of their experiences into classroom discussions, it eliminates the possibility that we can function as all-knowing, silent interrogators. But most professors must practice being vulnerable in the classroom, being wholly present in mind, body, and spirit.[32]

This means that our responsibility is to show up for our students with openness and gentleness. My students know *a lot* about how and what I practice. During the hybrid fall 2020 semester, I even made several videos of myself practicing, demonstrating that (a) I practice what I preach, (b) it works, (c) I'm not perfect, and (d) sometimes practicing is still messy for me, as it is for everyone. My students also know about my ADHD because it colors the way that I see things and process information. When I'm solving a problem,

I need to look away and limit how much sensory input is coming my way so that I can think more clearly. I sometimes need to take a deep breath before making technical suggestions because my brain gives me numerous ideas at once, and I need to filter them in real time. These behaviors might seem odd or off-putting without context. However, I'm very intentional about what I share with my students and *why*. I never ask students to do emotional labor on my behalf. They are not responsible for taking care of me, and I don't work out my feelings on them. When I share information with my students, it's because I think it can be of benefit to them. Demonstrating how a smart person with a neurodivergent brain functions in the workplace can be informative for them. Modeling healthy amounts of disclosure and good boundaries is another form of teaching.

5. Empowerment, Voice, and Choice

From our colleagues at ASHA:[33]

> H. Individuals shall obtain informed consent from the persons they serve about the nature and possible risks and effects of services provided, technology employed, and products dispensed.

The concept of informed consent in voice care feels like an important addition to the twenty-first-century voice teacher. What does your student want to sound like? What styles of music would they like to sing? If they are enrolled in a degree-granting program from an institution of higher education, how can you meet their needs while also ensuring that they are making timely academic progress? In the late 1990s, I entered college hoping to major in voice. I told the audition panel, "I want to teach singing, but first I want to learn everything there is to know about it." They asked me about my experience as a soloist (none) and my history of voice lessons (none) and suggested that I enroll in the music education track. This was sound academic advice at the time, because clearly, I had no idea what I was doing, and it was much easier to switch out of music ed (after three semesters) than it would have been to move into that incredibly packed major if I chose it several semesters down the line. I grew up listening to the radio and singing musicals. This is what I knew about singing. And suddenly I was (very appropriately) singing Purcell and Schumann and opera arias. Suddenly I found myself consumed with the pursuit of opera, considering master's programs that might put me on an imaginary fast-track to opera success (whatever that means), completely forgetting the music that had shaped my identity, and never asking myself what I wanted to do with my voice. I have only appreciation and respect for those early teachers, who gave me excellent repertoire and exposed me to a world of music I had never considered and thought I didn't like, but it wasn't until the second year of my doctoral studies (thirteen years later) that I really asked myself why I started singing in the first place and what I might like to do with my skills and training. This mindset is already shifting in academia, and more programs are adapting to provide students with an array of experiences and skills that empower them to make their own choices about how their art fits into their vision for life.

> J. Individuals shall accurately represent the intended purpose of a service, product, or research endeavor

Do your students know the purpose of every exercise you use in the studio? *Why* do we ask them to do composer research, and why do we require them to perform onstage? Can you reasonably justify the elements of your curriculum? If not, this is worthy of serious consideration within your department. At both universities where I've taught, musical theater majors are required to work on a classical selection each semester. This is often not their favorite curricular element, and some need a lot of support and external motivation to get this work done. The reasoning is not at all that classical technique is inherently "healthy," and if this is your logic you will have a very difficult time bringing students on board. I refer to this work as "vocal excavation," helping students to explore all of the things that their voices can do. For this reason, your classical majors should also be exploring musical theater repertoire, but only if they are required to experiment with stylistically appropriate technique. Does every coloratura soprano need to become a belter? Absolutely not. But all of your students should develop awareness of and comfort with every facet of their voices.

> K. Individuals who hold the Certificate of Clinical Competence shall evaluate the effectiveness of services provided, technology employed, and products dispensed, and they shall provide services or dispense products only when benefit can reasonably be expected.

Are your methods working? All teachers would do well to engage in rigorous self-reflection around their teaching practices. I tell all my students that my goal is to become obsolete; I want to teach them in such a way that they gain confidence in their problem-solving abilities, and a wide array of tools to help them meet the vocal challenges they will encounter. The studio conversations I have with my juniors and seniors are vastly different from the ones that occur with my first-year students. Sometimes students get "stuck" in their development and seem to plateau for several weeks, or an entire semester. When this happens, I look back through my notes to remind myself what we've discussed, what exercises we've explored, and how the student processed that information when given. Sometimes, all that's needed is a review of a big fundamental topic like breathing or alignment. In these instances, I'll go all the way back to the basics and watch the student closely as we discuss. I often ask if the information we're discussing conflicts with something else they've been taught, and openly discussing two different sets of instructions can be enough to clear the obstacles. Sometimes I need to ask the student why they think we're stuck. Their answers are usually informative and insightful.

6. Humility + Responsiveness to Cultural, Historical, and Gender Issues

From the APA Code of Ethics:[34]

> Principle E: Respect for People's Rights and Dignity
> Psychologists respect the dignity and worth of all people, and the rights of individuals to privacy, confidentiality, and self-determination. . . . Psychologists are aware of and respect cultural, individual, and role differences, including those based on age, gender, gender identity, race, ethnicity, culture, national origin, religion, sexual orientation, disability, language, and socioeconomic status, and consider these factors when working with members of such groups. Psychologists try to eliminate the effect on their work of biases based on those factors, and they do not knowingly participate in or condone activities of others based upon such prejudices.

Eliminating our biases is a crucial component of any helping profession. For teachers in white bodies, it is imperative to recognize that the lived experiences of Black and Indigenous People of Color (BIPOC) are different from your own. For cisgendered individuals, you must be aware that lived experience will vary for nonbinary, gender nonconforming, and transgender singers. This is a process that will take work, but is essential to decolonizing voice study, the opera industry, classical music, and music education. More on examining biases appears in chapters 9 and 10.

Things We Can Ethically Do

Consistency, Predictability, Clarity of Expectations[35]

Hopefully readers will find it comforting that you can contribute to healing simply by doing the things that you do every day. Traumatic events often arise quickly and overwhelm biological systems, so the consistency of regular lessons times, communicating absences well in advance, and structuring ongoing lessons in a similar way can help singers' nervous systems settle over time because they know what to expect, and can anticipate the level of sympathetic arousal that typically occurs in the course of your work together.

Challenge and Agency

> *Children and adults alike need to experience how rewarding it is to work at the edge of their abilities. Resilience is the product of agency: knowing that what you do can make a difference.*
>
> —Bessel van der Kolk[36]

Occasionally teachers want to push back against the idea of developing a trauma-informed approach, because they think that compassion equals coddling, and that by listening to our students and holding space for messy things, we will somehow be lowering our standards. If you were a calculus teacher and you found out on the first day of school that none of your students could add, I'd like to think that, rather than plowing ahead with advanced equations, you would find a way to help your students gain the skills necessary for success in your class. Many of our students come to us without the emotional skills necessary to interpret poetry and theatrical plot lines. Some of them are unprepared to work one-on-one in a studio with a person in a position of authority. Some of them live with depression, anxiety, shame, and/or PTSD. It's short sighted of us to expect them to do the equivalent of high-level musical calculus without tending to this gap in skills. And as we've mentioned, resilience skills come *after* safety is established. True, some of my singers take a little longer than others to settle into the studio and our working relationship, but when they find inner stability, they usually progress further than I would have imagined.

Developing a Sense of Self-Awareness

In *The Body Keeps the Score*, van der Kolk reports that the neuroscientist Joseph LeDoux and his colleagues have shown that "the only way we can consciously access the emotional brain is through self-awareness, i.e. by activating the medial prefrontal cortex, the part of the brain that notices what is going on inside us and thus allows us to feel what we're feeling."[37] He goes on to explain that a relationship with the body helps survivors to feel a sense of agency or control. This makes sense in the context of someone who is frequently and unpredictably beset with flashbacks, nightmares, recurring memories, or painful physical sensations. If one can cultivate an awareness of their physical form, it begins to create stable ground from which they can notice these symptoms without becoming engulfed by them. By definition, a sense of embodiment is the very opposite of dissociation, a common response to the overwhelm of trauma symptoms.[38] As van der Kolk explains, "The first step is to allow your mind to focus on your sensations and notice how, in contrast to the timeless, ever-present experience of trauma, physical sensations are transient and respond to slight shifts in body position, changes in breathing, and shifts in thinking."[39] As we discussed in chapter 1, the hypervigilance that many singers experience can lead to muscular constriction and tension throughout the body. This can sometimes lead to persistent defensiveness until someone is able to let their guard down when they perceive that they are safe.[40]

Van der Kolk explains that in his practice, helping patients to first notice, and then describe the sensations in their bodies is where the road to healing begins. He cautions us that what we are looking for are "not emotions such as anger or anxiety or fear but the physical sensations behind the emotions: pressure, heat, muscular tension, caving in, feeling hollow, and so on."[41] After a basic awareness of proprioception has developed, he then helps patients to become aware of breath, gestures, and movements, just as we do in vocal training as we help students to notice their habitual patterns of movement and make conscious choices about whether or not they serve the expressive vision of a piece or character. As van der Kolk explains, "Only by getting in touch with your body, by connecting viscerally with yourself, can you regain a sense of who you are, your priorities and values."[42]

The following exercises are adapted from Peter Levine's *Waking the Tiger*.[43]

Phase One: Proprioception

As Levine explains, "Learning to work with the felt sense may be challenging. Part of the dynamic of trauma is that it cuts us off from our internal experience as a way of protecting our organisms from sensations and emotions that could be overwhelming."[44] While ideally singers will cultivate a deep relationship with their bodies as a result of their training, it is important for teachers to know how to plant the seeds of awareness in a slow and methodical way.

When a student arrives in your studio, allow some time at the beginning of each lesson for landing in the body. It's most useful to engage in this exercise together so that the student doesn't end up feeling overly vulnerable as you watch them explore.

Begin at the top of the head and knead or tap on your skull to bring your complete awareness to the top of the head via external sensations. What does that area feel like? It may feel blank, numb, cold, tingly, disconnected; welcome any description available to your singer. Next, move to the back of the head. From there, progress to the muscles of the neck, shoulders, upper arms, forearms, and hands. You might choose to do this with all your beginning students to create a foundation for the other finely detailed body work you will do as you build skill.

Phase Two: The Felt Sense

Once a student has developed a beginning awareness of physical sensations and has some level of comfort in noticing sensation, you can begin to work together on what Levine calls "the felt sense."

Before the lesson begins, invite your student to become as comfortable as possible. Invite them to feel the contact they are making with the chair or the floor that is supporting them. Next, invite them to perceive whatever they can about the sensations of their skin: Can they feel clothing making contact with the skin? Can they perceive temperature or feel the movement of air? What sensations can you feel?

The point is not to change or control anything, but simply to notice what is happening in this exact moment. Give your student the choice of reporting their findings to you, or simply tracking them internally. The exercise is not designed to be performative and is in service of the student's developing skill.

I refer to both of these exercises as "landing," and along with a verbal check-in, they are foundational to every lesson. I have found that it's more specific than the nebulous idea of "grounding," which means different things in different modalities. If we ask students to "ground" without establishing a procedure, we can't really be sure of what they're doing. In this way, we methodically provide the tools necessary for singers to cultivate embodied singing.

Sound as a Regulating Stimulus

In *My Grandmother's Hands*, Resmaa Menakem introduces several sound exercises that voice practitioners could use at the start of any lesson.

Humming—take a few mindful breaths, and after the fourth or fifth, hum a long, comfortable tone until the end of the breath. Do this for two to three minutes, and then pause to notice what is happening in your body. Without doing anything else, notice what has changed, what's the same, and what sensations or thoughts are arising.[45]

Buzzing—begin as above but create a buzzing sound as you exhale (super bonus: this buzzing sound is also an example of a semi-occluded vocal tract exercise, meaning that it has technical applications as well). Sustain it as long as you can without forcing or constricting.[46]

Breathe, ground, and resource—take a few deep breaths and become aware of your body. Imagine a person, place, animal, or whatever that makes you feel safe and secure. Imagine that it's with you right now. Let yourself experience this safety and security for one to two minutes. Afterward, notice what you are feeling in your body.[47]

Experimenting with Emotional States

As a teacher of the performing arts, I was delighted to see Bessel van der Kolk advocating participation in theater as an indirect avenue of healing in *The Body Keeps the Score*. Many arts advocates repeat lofty platitudes about the healing power of the arts, but it was supremely validating to have a renowned researcher and medical professional bolster these claims based on his clinical experience of almost seventy years. He recounts that for many survivors the idea of feeling deep or intense emotions is frightening. In some cases, the last time that someone felt heightened emotions was during a traumatic experience, and so they may assume that any emotional response will be overwhelming. Some may have experienced that emotions lead to a loss of control. One benefit of engaging in the performing arts for survivors is that "theater is about embodying emotions, giving voice to them, becoming rhythmically engaged, taking on and embodying different roles."[48] This is also what happens when we give singers the opportunity to sing a variety of repertoire representing a wide array of voices and emotional states. Paul Griffin runs the Possibility Project in New York City, and both are featured in *The Body Keeps the Score*, where van der Kolk highlights the power of theater to help survivors embody and transform their pain. The Possibility Project "empowers young people to share their stories, transform their lives and impact their communities through writing, producing, and performing their own shows on the issues that matter to them the most."[49]

Griffin explains that

> [t]he job of any director [or performing arts teacher], like that of any therapist, is to slow things down so the actors can establish a relationship with themselves, with their bodies. Theater offers a unique way to access a full range of emotions and physical sensations that not only put them in touch with the habitual "set" of their bodies, but also let them explore alternative ways of engaging with life.[50]

Exploring Meta-Therapy (aka the "It" Factor)

In 1974, researcher David F. Ricks coined the term "supershrink" to describe therapists of an exceptional caliber. His study involved tracking long-term results for a group of adolescents categorized as "highly disturbed." When these same people were examined as adults, Ricks found that one group had far better outcomes overall, and they were all treated by the same therapist. Meanwhile, a group of people treated by a different clinician demonstrated "alarmingly poor adjustments as adults."[51] In 2005, Bruce Wampold and Jeb Brown conducted an even larger survey including 581 licensed providers and found that "clients of the best therapists in the sample improved at a rate at least 50 percent higher and dropped out at a rate at least 50 percent lower than those assigned to the worst clinicians in the sample."[52] Wampold and Brown also found that in cases where psychotropic medications were combined with therapy, the effectiveness of the medications depended on the quality of the therapist. Medications were found to be ten times more effective for patients working with the best therapists, and among those working with the worst therapists, medications made almost no difference, leading Wampold and Brown to summarize that "the catalyst is the clinician."

Practitioners are now investigating how these findings map onto voice care, most notably in the 2021 article "Mapping Meta-Therapy Interventions onto the Rehabilitation Treatment," written by Leah B. Helou and colleagues, published in *Seminars in Speech and Language*.[53] That paper acknowledges that "multiple fields of treatment that rely upon behavior change have widely accepted that the patient's perception of the clinician's warmth, empathy, and trust is a key driver of patient outcomes."[54] In addition, the authors note that psychological factors "such as stress, affect, and self-efficacy can play out in vocal subsystems and in voice itself."[55] Helou and colleagues explain that "high degrees of clinician empathy" may help establish the trust necessary for a patient to be honest and share information related to their voice disorder, and the patient's relationship with their own voice. The authors note that "it seems apparent" that variations in word choice and terminology, use of analogies, and explaining the "why" of specified exercises has "the potential to impact outcomes, above and beyond the specific contributions of classical direct and indirect therapy techniques."

All this is to say that some voice teachers hide behind the phrase "scope of practice" as a way to avoid contact with the more human elements of learning to sing. What research from psychology and voice therapy is telling us is that the people we work with *know* when we are not empathetic to their situations as learners, developing artists, and humans. Truth: a voice teacher without medical training may not proclaim to offer "vocal rehabilitation." Truth: voice teachers are not therapists. But I argue that the line between "I'm not a therapist" and "I will not discuss emotion in a lesson" is much larger than many voice teachers imagine. We now have a growing body of studies illustrating improved outcomes when people perceive warmth, care, and empathy from their providers. Listening is in the voice teacher's scope of practice. To put it another way, as I like to remind my students, "voice teachers are people too."

If we put up impenetrable walls around emotional content, we run the risk of re-traumatizing singers in a game that Elisa Monti refers to as "the trauma hot potato." Someone expresses their discomfort, or the truth about their lived experience, and if the teacher becomes reactive or uncomfortable, the singer gets the message that this expression of their humanity is not welcome. That lack of welcome can make a person carrying trauma feel isolated and/or ashamed for "sharing too much" or "being too emotional." When we can't hold space for singers' humanity and rush to toss the hot potato to someone else, we risk unconsciously communicating to a singer that we do not support them, and we are not willing to witness all of who they are. Chapter 8 addresses tools and practices for teachers to expand this capacity within themselves.

Notes

1. Bessel A. Van der Kolk, *The Body Keeps the Score: Brain Mind and Body in the Healing of Trauma* (New York: Penguin Books, 2015), 354.
2. "What Is Trauma-Informed Care?" Trauma-Informed Care Inplementation Resource Center, https://www.traumainformedcare.chcs.org/what-is-trauma-informed-care/.
3. Van der Kolk, *The Body Keeps the Score*, 223.
4. Ibid., 224.
5. Ibid., 127.
6. Ibid., 214.
7. American Speech-Language-Hearing Association. (2005). *The Role of the Speech-Language Pathologist, the Teacher of Singing, and the Speaking Voice Trainer in Voice Habilitation* [Technical Report]. Available from https://www.asha.org/policy/tr2005-00147/.
8. Marina Gilman, John Nix, and Edie Hapner, "The Speech Pathologist, the Singing Teacher, and the Singing Voice Specialist: Where's the Line?" *Journal of Singing* 67, no. 2 (November/December 2010): 171–78.
9. The Nationa Center for Voice and Speech, "Symposium on Specialty Training in Vocal Health: Summary Report," April 25–26, Salt Lake City, Utah, https://archive.ncvs.org/STVH_Summary_Report_2013.pdf
10. Pan American Vocology Association, "History," https://pavavocology.org/History.
11. "SAMHSA's Concept of Trauma and Guidance for a Trauma-Informed Approach," Youth.Gov, https://youth.gov/feature-article/samhsas-concept-trauma-and-guidance-trauma-informed-approach.

12. National Association of Teachers of Singing (NATS), "Code of Ethics," https://www.nats.org/code-of-ethics.html.
13. https://motivationalinterviewing.org/understanding-motivational-interviewing
14. https://inte.asha.org/siteassets/publications/et2016-00342.pdf
15. Van der Kolk, *The Body Keeps the* Score, 270–71.
16. SAMSHA (Substance Abuse and Mental Health Services Administration), "Interagency Task Force for Trauma-Informed Care," https://www.samhsa.gov/trauma-informed-care.
17. Ibid.
18. American Psychological Association (APA), "Ethical Principles of Psychologists and Code of Conduct," https://www.apa.org/ethics/code/ethics-code-2017.pdf.
19. Van der Kolk, *The Body Keeps the Score*, 214.
20. Denise Clark Pope, Maureen Brown, and Sarah B. Miles, *Overloaded and Underprepared: Strategies for Stronger Schools and Healthy, Successful Kids* (San Francisco: Jossey-Bass, 2015), 136–37.
21. Pope, *Overloaded and Underprepared*, 191.
22. Brené Brown, *Dare to Lead: Brave Work, Tough Conversations, Whole Hearts* (New York: Random House, 2018), 36–37.
23. Lynn Eustis, *The Teacher's Ego: When Singers become Voice Teachers* (Chicago: GIA Publications, Inc., 2013), 95.
24. Mark A. Bryan, Catherine A. Allen, and Julia Cameron, *The Artist's Way at Work: Riding the Dragon* (New York: William Morrow, 1998), 131.
25. Bryan et al., *The Artist's Way at Work*, xxi.
26. Eloise Ristad, *A Soprano on Her Head: Right-Side-Up Reflections on Life and Other Performances* (Lafayette: Real People Press, 1981), 132–33.
27. Deb Dana, *Anchored: How to Befriend Your Nervous System Using Polyvagal Theory* (Boulder: Sounds True, 2021), 10–12.
28. Van der Kolk, *The Body Keeps the Score*, 81.
29. Ibid.
30. APA, "Ethical Principles of Psychologists and Code of Conduct."
31. Van der Kolk, *The Body Keeps the Score*, 209.
32. bell hooks, *Teaching to Transgress: Education as the Practice of Freedom* (New York: Routledge, 1994), 21.
33. American Speech-Language-Hearing Association (ASHA), "Code of Ethics," 2015, https://inte.asha.org/siteassets/publications/et2016-00342.pdf
34. APA, "Ethical Principles of Psychologists and Code of Conduct."
35. Van der Kolk, *The Body Keeps the Score*, 355.
36. Ibid., 357.
37. Ibid., 208.
38. Ibid., 333
39. Ibid., 210.
40. Ibid., 102–3.
41. Ibid., 103.
42. Ibid., 249.

43. Peter A. Levine and Ann Frederick, *Waking the Tiger: Healing Trauma: The Innate Capacity to Transform Overwhelming Experiences* (Berkeley: North Atlantic Books, 1997), 63, 68.

44. Levine and Frederick, *Waking the Tiger*, 73.

45. Resmaa Menakem, *My Grandmother's Hands: Racialized Trauma and the Pathway to Mending Our Hearts and Bodies* (Las Vegas: Central Recovery Press, 2017), 141–42.

46. Ibid., 143.

47. Ibid., 146.

48. Van der Kolk, *The Body Keeps the Score*, 337.

49. The Possibility Project, https://www.the-possibility-project.org/.

50. Van der Kolk, *The Body Keeps the Score*, 339.

51. Scott Miller, Mark Hubble, and Barry Duncan, "Psychotherapy Networker Clinical Guide: The Secrets of Supershrinks: Pathways to Clinical Excellence," http://scottdmiller.com/wp-content/uploads/2014/06/Supershrinks-Free-Report-1.pdf.

52. Ibid.

53. Leah B. Helou, Jackie L. Gartner-Schmidt, Edie R. Hapner, Sarah L. Schneider, and Jarrad H. Van Stan, "Mapping Meta-Therapy in Voice Interventions onto the Rehabilitation Treatment Specification System," in *Seminars in Speech and Language* 42, no. 1 (2021): 005-018 (Thieme Medical Publishers, Inc., 2021).

54. Ibid., 52–55.

55. Ibid., 44–46.

7

When Music Makes the Wound

Emily Jaworski Koriath

As I progressed through my training in trauma healing, I was struck by how many times singing, humming, and chanting, alone and with others, appears in the literature. As a person who was trained in Western classical music through the American educational system, this did not resonate at all with my lived experience. My lowest point occurred during my doctorate, in the same Alexander Technique class that launched my interest in trauma. An instrumentalist told the class, "Whenever I get nervous or stressed about an audition or a performance, I play [Henry Mancini's] 'Moon River.' It was the first song I ever learned to play, and it makes me remember why I started in the first place." Our homework that week was to find our own personal "Moon River," a song that helped us drop in below the level of anxiety and conditioned thoughts and tap into a different sense of self. I experimented throughout the week, but ultimately discovered that at that point there was not a single thing I could sing in any genre that didn't fill me with frustration and self-loathing. I had developed extraordinary skill in noticing everything that I didn't like about my singing, but I still didn't have reliable tools to help me make the changes I was seeking.

Before we dive into what is sure to be a challenging conversation about pedagogical practices and the damage some singers have experienced, it is important for us to be aware that, as mentioned in chapter 5, not everything difficult is traumatic. As trauma becomes more prominent in our cultural awareness, there is a tendency for some to label any challenging dialogue or uncomfortable situation as trauma. While of course human systems vary, voice teachers have the unique opportunity to help singers learn to differentiate between what Resmaa Menakem refers to as "clean pain" and "dirty pain." Clean pain comes when we speak the truth in difficult circumstances, when we stand up for ourselves but get rejected anyway, when we hold boundaries in the face of pressure. As Menakem explains, clean pain is also what we experience as we heal and grow.

Dirty pain is what we experience when we pass our hurt on to others, when we silence ourselves so that others will stay comfortable, when we know abuse is occurring, but we say nothing. Menakem describes it best when he says, "When someone [has] unhealed trauma . . . [they] may try to push [their] trauma through another human being, by using violence, rage, coercion, betrayal, or emotional abuse. This only increases the . . . pain, while often creating trauma in the other person as well."[1] While we'll discuss clean and dirty pain in the context of the teacher's well-being in chapter 8, it's important to consider the popular adage that "hurt people hurt people," meaning that in many cases the root cause of an abusive studio environment may derive from abuse that the teacher suffered in the course of their own development. This is by no means a blanket excuse for racism, sexism, fatphobia, verbal and emotional abuse, bullying, and the flagrant exploitation of singers by sexual predators in positions of power. Academia, classical music, and the world of opera are moving toward a point of reckoning as singers are reporting mistreatment more boldly in the wake of the #metoo movement and other cultural shifts. We'll return to the discussion of these systemic issues after investigating some common sources of pain that may not always signal traumatic treatment.

Perfectionism

Real art only comes when you are willing to be something other than perfect.

—Lynn Eustis[2]

Perfectionism among musicians (especially classical musicians) is rampant, and I expect that listing it in a section about challenges in the learning process will raise many a perfectly manicured eyebrow. This can be confusing, because as professional musicians, the working standard is indeed perfection. If you get hired to sing the soprano solos in Handel's *Messiah*, but you don't know all the notes, if you even survive the rehearsal process and make it to the gig without getting fired, you would never be hired again. However, this standard absolutely does *not* apply in the practice room, where we should be free to experiment and get things wrong and make ugly sounds on purpose to excavate something beautiful underneath. Outside of music-making, we're allowed to consider the fact that we are fully human, and therefore imperfect by definition.

After I got my first post-doctorate, full-time, tenure-track job, I was making myself sick with anxiety. I wanted to take impeccable notes and make meaningful contributions in department meetings; I wanted to assign relevant, interesting, pedagogically appropriate, slightly off-the-beaten-path repertoire to every student, and I wanted to prepare them perfectly (this part is still true). I wanted to find national-level performing gigs and prominent outlets for some sort of research I hadn't even thought of yet and get fit and healthy and cook great meals and save a lot of money and wear fashionable, well-made, and interesting clothes, and look professional but funky, and make the most of living in an interesting city with a surprising amount of fantastic restaurants and lots of things to do all the time. Do you see where this is going? My wonderful department chair developed a very helpful habit of reminding me (quite often) that I was not required to earn tenure in my first year. Or even my second year! Sometimes the advice was "You don't need to get tenure today."

In the middle of a panic attack in my office, I was lying on the floor clutching my stomach and thinking that it was TOO HARD to have to be good at everything. It wasn't until later that I realized that yes, there are times in my life when I am required to be perfect, namely, the first rehearsal with the orchestra when there is no room for error. On closer examination, that only means that I know my material so well that I can focus on making music with the conductor and the orchestra. I might miss a cue, or misinterpret a tempo change, but these are the normal "getting to know you" bumps in the road on the way to performance. I had let something that was true only part of the time become the way that I approached everything, and it was causing me enormous anxiety. I hid all this behind a very calm demeanor because I needed everyone to think that I was smart, capable, put together, and always receptive, even in the face of challenges. Only as I continued my research in trauma did I realize that this approach was an overreaction to circumstances in my development. I was using this perfectionism as a shield, and a masking behavior for my ADHD. If we are treating *ourselves* this way, what are we modeling for our students? Do our unattainable standards apply to them, too? I worked with a student who lost their mother early in high school. Their dad remarried, and when the families blended, my student was the oldest of the children still living at home and was labeled "the easy one" compared to their younger and less independent new siblings. They continued to function more or less autonomously, but behind every decision was tremendous self-doubt, and a fear that if they needed help or clarification that it was too much for other people to be bothered with. This student needed a lot of reassurance and eventually got in the habit of texting me things like "Help, how do I quit this choir without making them hate me?"

No matter its source, perfectionism is correlated with depression, anxiety, addiction, and missed opportunities.[3] Its presence and the corresponding fear of failure and of making mistakes keeps students from taking creative risks and finding expressive freedom. Van der Kolk explains:

> As long as [someone's] map of the world is based on trauma, abuse, and neglect, people are likely to seek shortcuts to oblivion. Anticipating rejection, ridicule, and deprivation, they are reluctant to try out new options, certain that these will lead to failure. This lack of experimentation traps people in a matrix of fear, isolation, and scarcity where it is impossible to welcome the very experiences that might change their basic worldview.[4]

While we want our students to be musically excellent (an example of clean pain), that doesn't need to come at the expense of their humanity (dirty pain). We can teach them how to prepare rigorously. In the same season that I was recovering from a vocal injury, I sang Respighi's *Laud to the Nativity* with a choir that I knew and loved. I was righting my vocal ship, and I was making good progress in my recovery. I had also learned that I had to sing with my most excellent technique all the time to be successful in that state. One sloppy breath would literally cause me pain and interfere with my vocal function. The choir's conductor, Kristofer Johnson, sent the choir to their places with the reminder "Precision and joy! Precision and joy!" and that mantra resonated with me deeply. I could find joy in the performance by concentrating on critical details that would lead to my best possible work under the circumstances. We want our students to feel this way too—that technique is the path to greater satisfaction, not just another tool that makes us feel bad about ourselves. We can teach our students to be objective about their work; we can teach them deep listening and error detection so that if something does go wrong, they are the first to notice. None of that requires cruelty, shame, or blame. In *Dare to Lead*, Brené Brown writes that perfectionism isn't really about our motivation to do well, it's about trying to control the way we are perceived by others. This sets us up for continual failure because not only do we have no control over what others think of us, but also because perfection is not an attainable goal; perfection doesn't exist.[5] As I like to remind students, "perfection is incompatible with the human experience."

Shame

In 2016, psychologists Tanya Sariya and Teresa Lopez-Castro published a review of the available literature on the role of shame in the treatment of posttraumatic stress disorder (PTSD). In many cases, PTSD sufferers were not able to find relief of their symptoms, even after receiving care aligned with the highest therapeutic standards. Forty-seven studies met the established study criteria and provided substantial support for the association of shame with PTSD, as well as preliminary evidence that the treatment of underlying shame could be relevant to improved treatment outcomes.[6]

As Brown describes, we use our perfectionism as a shield in an attempt to hide our shame. A social worker and grounded theory researcher, Brown has dedicated her career to studying shame and its effects. Her first book, *I Thought It Was Just Me (But It Isn't)*, is a comprehensive deep dive on the causes of shame and how it shows up in our lives. In *Dare to Lead* she offers this brief summary on shame:[7]

1. We all have it. Shame is universal and one of the most primitive human emotions that we experience. The only people who don't experience shame are those who lack the capacity for empathy and human connections.
2. We're all afraid to talk about shame. Just the word is uncomfortable.
3. The less we talk about shame, the more control it has over our lives.

You might be able to give yourself a quick tutorial on physical symptoms of shame. Think of an embarrassing moment, close your eyes, and try to think as specifically as you can about how you felt. Did you get hot and flushed? Maybe you felt numb or tingly. Maybe you felt like you were being plunged into darkness, or that you were suddenly seeing everything unfold from a position slightly behind yourself. We manifest shame in many ways. Scientific evidence shows that the pain and isolation that we experience during moments of shame are as real as physical pain.[8] In moments of shame, we also employ strategies of disconnection. We feel unlovable, and we think that if people saw us in this state, all of our worst fears would come true. Singers with a complex trauma history deal with layers of shame.

When we are in the grip of shame, our interactions with others fall into one of three categories, as described by Brown.[9] Some of us default to behaviors categorized as "moving away": withdrawing physically or emotionally, hiding, or silencing ourselves. Others might try "moving toward" behaviors: trying to appease or please the other party . . . Stephen Porges talks about "moving toward" behaviors as a survival strategy when the vagus nerve is activated under extreme threat. You'll recall from chapter 2 that because the social engagement elements of our personalities are at the top of the vagal hierarchy, we often try to engage socially to mitigate threats. This is why, seemingly illogically, people may try to speak to someone holding them at gunpoint or trying to hurt them in some way. Our biological wiring tells us that if we are conversing pleasantly, we can keep danger at bay. That same wiring is activated in a shame response. Lastly, in the face of shame, some people will attempt to "move against" by trying to gain power over others. This explains why some people lash out verbally and try to use the shaming of another to fight their own shame.

Understanding shame gives us insights into common behaviors in the studio. When students are feeling shame, they may turn red, get stony faced, or tears might spring in the eyes. They may become silent or excessively verbal. Depending on trauma history, some of them may shut down completely and be unable to proceed. It's also important for educators to realize that some students will take people-pleasing behaviors to an extreme level in order to hide their true feelings about themselves. Many think that obtaining a certain level of achievement will somehow convince others of their worth. Sadly, in the world of classical music, some students begin to distinguish themselves due to an extreme adherence to instructor expectations. I have seen many singers bend over backward to attempt to predict what an audition panel will want to hear. I remember hearing a soprano say that audition season was the time for fake boobs, fake hair, fake nails, and a fake tan. We have unintentionally taught many singers that erasing themselves as individuals is the path to success in the opera industry.

If you correct a rhythm in a lesson and the student's reaction seems out of proportion to the situation, they may be awash in their shame response. Always proceed gently if you suspect that shame is in play. In these moments, *all people* feel the most alone, the most unworthy. We have an opportunity to name their shame, or at least acknowledge that something has ruptured. I'll invite a student to consider a quick walk down the hallway, or I'll offer to leave the room for a few minutes. If they feel it best to leave the lesson, I will honor their decision, and *always* check in later. Most importantly, check your own emotions about whatever is happening and prioritize the care of the student, who is still learning to navigate the personal elements of this work. Hopefully as the teacher, you've developed a sturdy support system if you need to process your experience with someone later. Remember that in many cases, the student's support system might not exist, or it might be in development and only consist of you. In order to maintain the emotional safety and trust required for deep emotional work, these ruptures must be repaired.

By understanding how shame functions in all of us, and how it appears in the studio, we can gain perspective and begin to recognize when we are experiencing shame. I've been practicing this for a while now and can say to my students, "Oh, I can feel how that brings a tear to my eye," or "I can feel myself struggling with that, and I just need a second to let that settle." I do this because I want to model healthy processing for them, and because I want them to be able to trust me. If I fall back on my perfectionist ways and try to appear unfazed and above it all, I'm unconsciously teaching them disconnection as a way of being. Would you be comfortable sharing your truest self with someone if you felt they weren't being honest with you? Shame is a universal human emotion. When we feel most alone, most unlovable, most unworthy, we are actually being most fully human, just like everyone else.

Mindset

The last major obstacle to discuss is *mindset*. According to psychologist Richard G. Tedeschi, the author of 2018's *Posttraumatic Growth*, trauma creates a rupture in our belief patterns and our understanding of the world. This is confusing and frightening and can often produce anxious and repetitive thinking.[10] After trauma occurs, it can be easy to think that we have been damaged in the process and will always remain so, but Tedeschi reports that "negative experiences can bring a recognition of personal strength, the exploration of new possibilities, improved relationships with others, a greater appreciation for life, and spiritual growth."[11]

Tedeschi's insights on posttraumatic growth tie into Stanford psychologist Carol Dweck's research on mindset, originally published in book form in 2006. Dweck explains that people fall into two categories: the fixed mindset and the growth mindset.

The *fixed mindset* is the belief that your qualities are carved in stone; you are the way you are, and you were born with a certain number of skills and qualities. You're good at some things and bad at some things, and those things will never change.[12] You may notice some resonance here with Tedeschi's insights about the ways our thinking patterns can get stuck in negative cycles in response to the upheaval of trauma. In Dweck's research, a fixed mindset can develop when we are frequently praised for being talented. Risk and effort are to be avoided because these are reserved for people who don't have your skills and "talents"; in other words, having to put in effort might reveal your inadequacies and show that you were not up to the task.[13] She goes on to explain that those with the fixed mindset think "Either you have the ability *or* you expend effort" because people with the fixed mindset think that effort is for those who don't have the ability, and if you have to work at something, you must not be good at it.[14] In the wake of trauma, it can be easy to develop a fixed mindset that is formed by our desire to keep things manageable for our psyche; we mistakenly believe that making fewer choices, taking fewer risks, and overall experiencing less might keep us safe.

Sadly, I have seen the fixed mindset in the studio often, usually within a student's first few weeks in school. Many of them are "big fish" in their small high school ponds. They are praised for their talent and sometimes are the only music major that their town has produced. They have promising entrance auditions, but as lessons begin, something feels "off." They are slow to make adjustments during exercises. Their repertoire doesn't seem to progress as you might expect. Frequently this is because they don't know how to practice. Not only do they not know how, but because of their fixed mindset, they think that they should not *need* to practice. After all, they are talented! If they were really as good as everyone says, they shouldn't *have to* practice. Practicing is only for people who are not as good. Practicing would be an admission that everyone who believed in them was wrong or that the student is really a fraud. Cue the shame response, as described above.

To me, mindset explains why music theory coursework has taken on such "make or break" significance for undergraduates. Many incoming students have been successful in their school music programs but have never had to do anything like theory before. For many, it's the first time they've had to do anything in the field of music that challenges them, and this is why some of them freak out; they've not encountered academic setbacks, and the prospect of this is so terrifying that they cannot see a way forward. Teachers might be tempted to dismiss these students as lazy or entitled when the true problem is that they have been protected from challenge up until this point. A keen understanding of mindset, whether it has arisen organically or as the result of trauma, gives us an opportunity to reach out to these students and help move them subtly toward the growth mindset before they quit. As van der Kolk explains, "If an organism is stuck in survival mode, its energies are focused on fighting off unseen enemies. . . . [A]s long as the mind is defending itself against invisible assaults, our closest bonds are threatened, along with our ability to imagine, play, learn, and pay attention to other people's needs."[15]

In the fall of 2020, I briefly introduced the concept of fixed mindset in a studio class. Even in our virtual gathering space, I could feel my students become very, very silent as they let the concept sink in.

On the other hand, "the *growth mindset* is based on the belief that your basic qualities are things you can cultivate through your efforts[;] . . . everyone can change and grow through application and experience."[16] In a poll Dweck conducted of 143 creativity researchers, there was wide agreement about the number-one ingredient in creative achievement. It was exactly the kind of perseverance and resilience produced by the growth mindset: "the love of challenge, belief in effort, [and] resilience in the face of setbacks."[17] The growth mindset allows people to value what they're doing *regardless of the outcome*.[18] As Tedeschi wrote for the Harvard Business Review, "to do any learning, one must be in the right frame of mind. That starts with managing negative emotions such as anxiety, guilt, and anger, which can be done by shifting the kind of thinking that leads to those feelings."[19]

Mindset at School

The good news is that Dweck's research has also shown that mindset is changeable. We can start by making sure that when we praise students, we are praising effort, not "talent." The way that we structure our feedback can help as well. Dweck explains:

> Children need honest and constructive feedback. If children are "protected" from it, they won't learn well. They will experience advice, coaching, and feedback as negative and undermining. Withholding constructive criticism does not help children's confidence; it harms their future.[20]

This can make for some rough times of transition, because those with a fixed mindset can view feedback as a threat, an insult, or an attack.[21] A teaching colleague told me about informing a student that they were not consistently singing in tune. It later got back to my colleague that this student reported to their friends that this feedback was "damaging." On the surface, this might sound like a bizarre, dramatic, or hilarious anecdote. What it really demonstrates is a perfect example of the fixed mindset in action. Singing in tune is a professional requirement; it's non-negotiable. In fact, I would argue that if you have students who sing out of tune and you *don't* tell them about it, *that* would constitute damaging behavior because we would be putting a stamp of approval on someone and sending them out into the world without adequate preparation. We need to know that many of our students view feedback this way, especially the ones who were known as high achievers in high school. When students get accustomed to being praised for being great, they may be set up to struggle in college. Many students think that any criticism means that the teacher hates them because, as van der Kolk explains, "If your amygdala goes into overdrive, you may become chronically scared that people hate you."[22] As teachers, we need to be aware of this phenomenon and sensitive to it, and look for signs that it's happening so that when we do provide feedback, we can try to do it in a way that students can hear. Truly, if my colleague's student wants to be a singer of any kind, they need to sing in tune. But it's also true that at least in that moment, they couldn't hear that as useful feedback; they heard it as abuse. This example highlights the fact that we need to teach our students how to hear criticism. Strategies around feedback appear later in this chapter.

I had a similar disorienting experience myself when I began my doctoral studies with Dr. Eustis. It was confusing to me that she had incredibly high standards but was not actually mean. She was truly, deeply supportive; but at first, I was defensive. My conditioning had led me to believe that high expectations are always accompanied by cruelty or callousness. I remember getting intensely frustrated in a lesson because I was trying *so hard* to incorporate new technical advice, but my brain and body were still not clicking together after a few months. I turned to Dr. E and asked, "Do you know that I'm trying really hard to do what you're asking me?" I wanted her to know that I was not trying to be resistant, and I did understand the concepts. I chose the clean pain of telling the deepest truth about what I was feeling, rather than the dirty pain of remaining frustrated in the lesson and shutting down. My teacher assured me that, of course she knew that I was trying, which was wildly reassuring to me. That was a defining moment for me as a learner because I stopped being afraid of disappointing my teacher, and I fully trusted her because she could *see* me. She knew I was working hard but encountering difficulty, and she knew why it was hard for me to incorporate new technical concepts as a thirty-something doctoral student with years of engrained muscle memory. She was prepared to be patient as new technical ideas took hold, but she also didn't stop insisting that the breaths I took were useful, that I sang real vowels, and that I remained mentally present while singing. There were a few similar breakthrough moments as my defensive walls came down, and I was eventually able to interact with her as she was, not as I projected her to be.

A few months into my program, someone asked me about Dr. Eustis and what it was like to study with her. I said, "I have never met a person with higher standards, *and* I have never met a person as supportive in helping you to reach those standards." At the time, I had no idea that I had just summed up the qualities of a growth-minded educator. Dweck explains that many teachers mistakenly think that in order to facilitate student success and feelings of confidence, they must lower their standards. Evidence suggests that this strategy doesn't work, and only creates students who feel entitled to lots of praise for very little effort. Conversely, if we raise standards or maintain high standards *without giving students the means of reaching them*, we are also setting them up for frustration and failure.[23] As we'll discuss next, the art is in telling the truth with kindness and understanding.

Feedback Skills

Without real conversations around feedback, there is less learning and more defensiveness.

—Brené Brown

In a profession where the goal is continued growth, and artists interact with numerous coaches, teachers, conductors, and colleagues at every turn, we know that our students will be presented with endless amounts of feedback around their work. Teachers should be skilled in the art of providing feedback for their students, and they should also provide their students with tools to filter the feedback they will inevitably receive from others. It's imperative that our feedback to students is clear, precise, and actionable. If a pitch is out of tune, say exactly that and offer some strategies before asking the student to try again. There's no need for personal criticisms or manipulative undertones to our comments. The student isn't a failure or a waste of your time if they're out of tune; no one sings out of tune on purpose or to annoy you. If a student is displaying a technical deficiency, they need your help, not your disdain. If we are engaging with students in a disparaging way on a regular basis, it's likely a reflection of the way that we were taught ourselves. To find a different approach to feedback, it may be helpful to process this for yourself. Can you remember a particular cutting comment aimed at you in your developmental stage as an artist? Be slow and gentle as you take a few deep breaths and remember as much as you can about that moment. Where were you? In a lesson, coaching, practice room, studio? How old were you at the time, and how did this criticism hurt you at that stage of your development? Now imagine that the recipient of that remark is your student. What would you say to them as the caring and compassionate teacher you are to help them process this moment of hurt?

By completing this exercise, either in thought or in writing, you give yourself a chance to process that pain so that you don't continue passing it on. You also have the opportunity to stretch your compassion to your students and feel what it feels like to imagine hurting them. None of us tries to hurt students intentionally, but we may not be aware of how much power we have to do just that.

In addition to making our own feedback kinder and more useful, we should also be teaching students how to filter the feedback they get from other, sometimes less careful, sources. We need to be able to hear criticism without activating our self-protective responses, so that we can stay vulnerable and courageous in our work. Brené Brown suggests that the ultimate goal is a skillful blend of listening and integrating feedback. We accomplish this by staying curious, staying calm, asking questions if something doesn't make sense, and avoiding defensiveness.[24]

It can be difficult in the moment to glean something useful from an observer's comment, especially if it is delivered in a way that brushes up against our sensitivities, but one of the worst things we do to ourselves is hold onto those comments and replay them over and over in our minds. You may recall that this is especially likely for your students who have developed an anxious attachment style. I still remember a judge's comment from a voice competition I competed in during my master's degree, scolding me for not wearing hosiery. Hopefully those days have passed and we're not doing that to people anymore, but at the time I found this so bizarre and unhelpful that I told everyone about it. I kept replaying that scene in my mind and every time I told the story, I gave this criticism more power. It was shaping my choices about what I would wear in auditions, but not in a helpful way. I felt an urge to be defiant and I got more focused on that than on engaging in preparations that would help me present stronger auditions. Why would someone comment on hosiery? In a ten-minute audition, was there nothing else that I did that was worthy of mention? Now I understand that this feedback had much more to do with whoever wrote it than it did with me. But at the time, I was desperate for approval and for reassurance that I was doing well. I wanted to keep getting better, and what I was really feeling was disappointment that my comment sheets weren't full of sweeping praise for me and my craft. If we're teaching our students well, we're helping them to find value in their work *regardless* of what others say. That makes it much easier to recognize the difference between feedback that has value and feedback that they can appreciate and release.

Paths to Trauma in the Studio

Most harm in vocal training occurs when singers are seen as voices or products and not as people. Music educator and researcher Freya Larman-Ivens writes that professional singers are "often heard to talk about 'the voice' as opposed to 'my voice,' implying that they perceive the voice as an instrument that is not exactly and entirely a part of them."[25] Unfortunately, this imagined separation can lead some teachers to relentlessly criticize "a voice," forgetting that it belongs to a *person*. Sometimes our curiosity and fascination with a vocal instrument leads us to overlook how our questions and observations might be perceived by a singer. I once watched a master class where two teachers peered into the open mouth of a singer with a flashlight to determine the position of the singer's soft palate. In that moment I thought to myself, "How is that singer feeling at this moment?" and "What are we doing here?"

Occasionally a teacher launches a handful of successful pupils into the world using a particular set of methods, and then becomes convinced that this is "The Way," as though there is only one path. The deeper a teacher becomes entrenched in a certain method or overall approach, the more tempting it becomes to think that when these same methods fail to produce results in a student, that it must be that student's fault. They are simply not as talented or not as smart as your former pupils. As pedagogue William Sauerland writes in *Queering Vocal Pedagogy*, it is easy to "imagine a voice teacher who unintentionally, but nonetheless systematically, stifles or dismisses a singer through their preconceived notions of what the student's goals should be."[26] What this fictional teacher has failed to consider is that every human being is different. While there are some universal truths about human anatomy and the physics of sound, learning is a complex task governed by innumerable factors. Something as simple as the time of day can limit your student's capacity to take in new information, to take risks, and to synthesize the learning that takes place over the course of the semester. A skilled teacher will not only understand which elements of the art of singing are universal and which are subjective but will also have a myriad of ways to explain concepts and be unafraid of engaging in dialogue with students about how they may learn best. Lynn Helding's outstanding book *The Musician's Mind* should be required reading for every teacher. We are responsible not only for teaching excellent content, but for teaching that material in a way that facilitates student learning. Your students may not yet know how optimal practicing works, or even *what* they should be practicing. This isn't their fault, and they are not doing it to irritate you. There is a disconnect in learning that teachers can remedy.

Gender in Voice Study

As Sauerland summarizes in *Queering Vocal Pedagogy,* voice study has some deeply entrenched practices that reinforce gender binary and heteronormativity. Consider how many songs in treble voice anthologies are settings of texts about flowers and lullabies, and how many tenor/baritone/bass anthologies include songs about adventure or shipmates. How often in ensembles or musical theater auditions are singers grouped as "men" and "women"? While this choice of language may seem innocuous, conversations with trans and gender-nonconforming singers reveal that this practice can feel isolating, as though there is no place in vocal music for someone who doesn't easily fit into a specific category. I had a glimpse of what this kind of othering feels like early in my training. While my voice was still developing (and disconnected from my body), I had a whistle register and fast coloratura (mostly because my voice lacked substance). I sang soubrette rep, or music for light soprano from the operatic repertoire. In some circles, these types of characters are referred to "-inas and -ettas;" characters with names like Despina, Norina, Giulietta who were mostly lovely ingenues. I am nearly six feet tall with an athletic frame, and even when I started to find repertoire that suited my voice well, I was repeatedly told that I would never be hired for these types of roles. I have never identified as stereotypically "female," so singing about how pretty I am was never interesting to me. But if my body didn't match the repertoire that I was singing best, what was I supposed to do? This also explains my utter delight at finding out that I am really a mezzo. I always describe that moment like a light shining down from heaven, and I remember thinking, "Finally! I can play boys! My body makes sense now!" I want to make clear that I am in no way equating my mild discomfort with the lived experience of trans and genderqueer singers, just that having lived though this feeling of not fitting made me deeply empathetic to what singing could feel like for others whose gender identities don't match the sound that they produce, or who are required to sing gendered songs with specific pronouns about "he" characters or "she" characters that don't align with the singer's authentic self. Neither should we assume that all trans singers want to sing songs about being trans, or that all LGBTQ+ singers want to sing only the music of gay characters or gay poets.

Race and Voice

In an article for *Postmodern Culture*, Nina Sun Eidsheim described her exploration of why certain race-based thoughts about singing still persist and are reproduced, despite a distinct lack of scientific evidence to support those myths. Eidsheim explained that notions of "white sound" and "Black sound" still exist for many voice professionals, and many singing teachers assert that they can discern a singer's race just by listening.[27] In music education research, extensive discussion has been going on for years among researchers striving to decolonize the music classroom and to place value on non-Western music as equally valid forms of art worthy of study. A student of color recently related a conversation they had with a peer about performing on Broadway. The two singers shrugged their shoulders and decided they just needed to hope that *Hamilton* was still running when they graduate. I have had students ask me to help them find music by composers who share their ethnicity, and I know classical musicians of color who just want to make music and do not want to be assigned the role of advocate for their entire race. As voice professionals, we should not make assumptions about what kinds of music singers are interested in based on their visible identities. As we work to expand the standard vocal repertoire to include more historically marginalized composers, *all* of our students should be singing music by composers of color, and by women, and by trans and genderqueer composers. I could never hope to distill all of the complexities of race and voice in a simple paragraph, and I recognize that the topic of race and voice have already been explored expertly in several important texts. Scholar Naomi André published *Black Opera: History, Power, Engagement* in 2018, and served as the editor for 2014's *Blackness in Opera*, deeply fertile ground for voice teachers to begin (or continue) their own study on race and voice.

As discussed in chapter 6, a good teacher will consider it a priority to continue developing expertise in their work and pursuing multiple perspectives. What do teachers of pop music have to say about resonance and diction that could apply to your singers in other genres? What can you learn about anatomy from exploring a Rolfing series, or ancient Chinese medicine? Part of what makes a highly skilled teacher is the ability to weave together empirical knowledge and lived experience. Taking your technical knowledge for a walk through other related areas will help you focus your pedagogy while also broadening it. Each of our students come to us with a completely singular set of skills and experiences. A fantastic teacher will find ways to honor this and work with each singer to determine how the teacher's expertise can support the singer on their own musical and personal path.

Lastly, as mentioned earlier in this text, some teachers in academia still operate under the assumption that every singer they meet should be preparing for an operatic career. Dana Lynne Varga, soprano, pedagogue, and founder of the Empowered Musician refers to this as the *opera pipeline*, where students are taught that they need to win specific competitions and participate in certain young artist programs (YAPs), and that by following one specific order of operations, one may magically find oneself at the top of the operatic food chain. While this may have been true for an extraordinarily small group of people at one point in time, the reality is that today's operatic marketplace is absolutely flooded with singers of high quality with not enough jobs to go around. This is especially damaging for sopranos, who are told repeatedly that they are "a dime a dozen" and that any mistake or perceived flaw means that there are a hundred other singers in line to take their place. By inculcating this mindset into continuing cohorts of singers, we start to cultivate a cutthroat mentality and perpetuate the idea that singers are competing against each other for jobs, for attention, for their very livelihoods. There is a rampant zero-sum mindset that says that someone else's success means yet another opportunity that you have missed. As a beloved colleague told me after I failed to advance to the finals of a competition that I held near and dear to my heart, "[T]here are as many ways to be a singer as there are people who want to sing." When we train students to think that success looks one very particular way, then anything else they accomplish, no matter how great, may be perceived as "less than," even if it comes from the student's deepest desires. We accidentally train singers that if they don't "make it" (whatever that means), then it's their fault.

The time of verbally abusing students for what the teacher perceives as "their own good" must die immediately. Fear is not a motivational technique. It is well documented that when learners are experiencing fear, anxiety, or anger, their capacity for reason decreases,[28] and yet some teachers still insist on demeaning their students for not practicing enough, telling them that they simply "don't want it enough," or that if they really cared about being a singer, then they would (insert demand of teacher's choice). As discussed in chapter 1, ongoing nervous system activation leads to muscular tension and the release of stress hormones in the body. This is not the fertile ground from which great artistry is cultivated. You cannot berate someone into expressivity. Don't tell your students they won't make it and they should quit. You absolutely can give them a realistic assessment of where they may be in relation to their goals (and remember, those are *the student's* goals; more in chapter 9), but even this can be done with kindness and understanding. For example, I have heard teachers say things along the lines of "Well, you'll certainly never make it to the Met singing like that!" And while the underlying sentiment may be true, what the student hears is a trusted figure telling them that they are not good enough? It would be much more productive to sit down with this singer and have an in-depth conversation. For example, the teacher can begin by saying, "I'd like to talk about how your lessons are going, especially as you think of your future goals." It's most productive to plant this seed and then schedule the conversation for a future time, so the singer has an opportunity to reflect on how things are progressing. As a neurodivergent singer, it's very difficult for me to change the direction of my thinking quickly. If I'm trying to learn and thinking deeply about French vowels but then you ask me about my future plans, I may go blank, be unable to communicate my thoughts or not even remember that I have future plans. Several hours later, my brain will have produced a very detailed map of all my thoughts and concerns. Many people need time to think and process before engaging in conversations in-depth.

Our students come to us because they love singing. Our job is to educate them about the many facets of the performing arts industry and the realities of art as a profession, and to provide them with the tools to pursue whatever version of art making that correlates to their vision of a rich and fulfilling life. The following instructions are derived from real singers' stories about the harm they encountered in their training. Never tell a student you hate their voice. Never tell a student that if they can't sing like you do that they should quit. Never tell them that they are too fat. Don't tell them they are too tall or too short. Don't yell at them for making mistakes. Don't force them onto a path that they're not interested in. Don't try to live vicariously through them. Never, ever, ever, ever tell a student that they won't be cast because they're Black. Don't mock their speech impediment or accent. Don't assume they are lazy if something isn't working the way you expect it to.

Notes

1. Resmaa Menakem, *My Grandmother's Hands: Racialized Trauma and the Pathway to Mending Our Hearts and Bodies* (Las Vegas: Central Recovery Press, 2017), 54.

2. Lynn Eustis, *The Singer's Ego: Finding Balance between Music and Life: A Guide for Singers and Those Who Teach and Work with Singers* (Chicago: GIA Publications, Inc., 2005), 14.

3. Brené Brown, *Dare to Lead: Brave Work, Tough Conversations, Whole Hearts* (New York: Random House, 2018), 79.

4. Bessel A. Van der Kolk, *The Body Keeps the Score: Brain Mind and Body in the Healing of Trauma* (New York: Penguin Books, 2015), 307.

5. Brown, *Dare to Lead,* 80.

6. Tanya Saraiya and Teresa Lopez-Castro, "Ashamed and Afraid: A Scoping Review of the Role of Shame in Post-Traumatic Stress Disorder (PTSD)," *Journal of Clinical Medicine* 5, no. 11 (2016): 94. doi:10.3390/jcm5110094.

7. Brown, *Dare to Lead*, 101–25.

8. Naomi Eisenberger, Matthew Lieberman, and Kipling Williams, "Does Rejection Hurt? An fMRI Study of Social Exclusion," *Science* (2003): 290–92. doi:10.1126/science.1089134.

9. Brown, *Dare to Lead*, 161.

10. Richard G. Tedeschi, "Growth After Trauma," *Harvard Business Review*, July-August 2020, .https://hbr.org/2020/07/growth-after-trauma. Accessed June 24, 2020

11. Ibid.

12. Carol Dweck, *Mindset: The New Psychology of Success* (New York: Ballantine Books, 2007), 6.

13. Dweck, *Mindset*, 10.

14. Ibid., 40.

15. Van der Kolk, *The Body Keeps the Score*, 76.

16. Dweck, *Mindset*, 7.

17. Ibid., 12.

18. Ibid., 48.

19. Tedeschi, "Growth After Trauma.

20. Dweck, *Mindset*, 182.

21. Ibid., 76.

22. Van der Kolk, *The Body Keeps the* Score, 69.

23. Dweck, *Mindset*, 193–94.

24. Brown, *Dare to Lead* 198–202.

25. As quoted in William Sauerland, *Queering Vocal Pedagogy: A Handbook for Teaching Trans and Genderqueer Singers and Fostering Gender-Affirming Spaces* (Lanham, MD: Rowman & Littlefield, 2022), 42.

26. Ibid., 21.

27. "The Micropolitics of Listening to Vocal Timbre," *Postmodern Culture: Journal of Interdisciplinary Thought on Contemporary Cultures* 24, no. 3 (May 2014): https://www.pomoculture.org/2017/09/09/the-micropolitics-of-listening-to-vocal-timbre/.

28. Van der Kolk, *The Body Keeps the* Score, 88.

III

A NEW WAY FORWARD

8

Finding Stable Ground

Emily Jaworski Koriath

The most important technique in trauma stewardship is learning to stay fully present in our experience, no matter how difficult.[1]

VOICE TEACHER AND MOVEMENT EXPERT SARAH WHITTEN offers us the following:

The human body is responsive and interactive with the environments it encounters. That means we are constantly in an exchange with the people and places around us. The body remembers through implicit and explicit memory. It also changes constantly and holds an immense amount of innate intelligence and wisdom.

When we encounter a singer in a lesson or coaching, we are meeting all of their memories and intelligence and they are responding and interacting with the environment of us and our studio. The intimate nature of vocal study means one of the top qualities a voice teacher can cultivate is the ability to be present. Presence allows us to observe what is happening with a singer AND what is happening in ourselves at the same time.

Being present means we are connected to and aware of our own experiences. We are committed to noticing when those experiences might trigger changes in our being. And, we are committed to engaging in practices that can pull us back into our body when something pulls us out.

The quality of our presence makes an enormous difference to the people we work with. The singing body is more apt to respond positively when it knows we are a safe place. This doesn't mean we are constantly perfectly attuned to ourself. It does mean we are able to [be] honest, kind, and compassionate with ourself about where we are at on any given day.

> Engaging in something as simple as a somatic snapshot before beginning our teaching day or in between sessions is a wonderful way to begin to cultivate our presence. You can try asking yourself three questions (and answer them honestly!) 1. How am I feeling today? 2. What are the sensations in my body right now and where are they located? 3. If my body could speak, what would it say to me right now?
>
> Sarah Whitten
MA Vocal Pedagogy
MM Vocal Performance
Movement for Trauma Certification
Integrative Somatic Trauma Therapy Certification

Teachers and Stress

Rupa Marya and Raj Patel, coauthors of *Inflamed: Deep Medicine and the Anatomy of Injustice*, offer a helpful, holistic definition of stress in terms of systems of the body. They write,

> Biologically speaking, stress is a state of real or perceived threat to homeostasis. It is provoked by psychological, environmental, and physiological stimuli that create a cascade of hormones, neurotransmitters, and cytokines working together to restore homeostasis. The stress response is a tightly choreographed interaction between the immune, endocrine, and nervous systems. It addresses actual or potential damage and is intimately integrated with the inflammation response.[2]

A biological mechanism known as the hypothalamic-pituitary-adrenal (HPA) axis works to mitigate the effects of stress on the body by regulating numerous internal processes such as metabolism, immune response, and activation of the nervous system.[3] The HPA axis and nervous system "together affect the executive, cognitive, fear, reward, and sleep/wake centers of the brain. They also impact the gastrointestinal, reproductive, cardiovascular, respiratory, immune, and endocrine systems."[4] Just like we discovered with heightened nervous system states, human organisms are not designed to remain in constant states of stress. To do so "leads to pathological manifestations, such as low-grade inflammation and decreased immune response in the face of viral infections."[5] Chronic stress makes us vulnerable to addiction and can decrease our impulse control. As Patel and Marya explain in *Inflamed*, the more chronic our stress becomes, the more maladaptive our behavior becomes.

"Chronic stress dampens activity in the prefrontal cortex—the part of the brain responsible for rational decision making and self-control—and heightens activity in the limbic system, which includes the amygdala, an ancient center of the brain that guides impulsive behavior."[6] We've discussed these brain areas before in relation to the body's response to trauma. While we are learning to monitor our students for signs of such distress, it will be crucial to take inventory of our own internal state.

In *Permission to Feel*, Marc Brackett of the Yale Center for Emotional Intelligence reports some alarming findings: 46 percent of teachers report high daily stress (tied with nurses for the highest rate among all jobs); 50 percent of employees across all fields are unengaged at work; and 13 percent are "miserable."[7] Forty percent of teachers leave the profession within five years, and in some communities the rate is as high as 30 percent annually. Seventy percent of the emotions that those surveyed feel each day are negative—mainly "frustrated," "overwhelmed," and "stressed." This is especially troubling because teachers who experience more negative emotions are also more likely to have sleep problems, anxiety, and depression, be burned out, and have greater intentions to leave the profession. And of course, these data were collected before COVID-19 and the "Great Resignation." But you don't need these numbers to tell you how you feel. If you suspect that you're burning out, you probably are. Just in case, there are some sneaky ways that our bodies and brains will let us know when we've had too much. As Laura van Dernoot Lipsky wrote in *Trauma Stewardship*, simmering anger was her cue that something was wrong. Actually, van Dernoot Lipsky acknowledges several times in the text that these clues let *her family* know that something was wrong; the author was not able to perceive her own distress without the support of others.

> Rather than acknowledge my own pain and helplessness in the face of things I could not control, I raged at the possible external causes. I sharpened my critique of systems and society. I became more dogmatic, opinionated, and intolerant of others' views than ever before. It never occurred to me that my anger might in part be functioning as a shield against what I was experiencing.[8]

The negative emotions we experience at work also have serious ramifications for our students: teachers who are stressed offer less information and praise, are less accepting of student ideas, and interact less frequently with students. The effects are clear: Brackett and his team surveyed twenty-two thousand high school students and asked them, "How do you feel each day in school?" Seventy-seven percent of collected responses were negative. The most common answers were "tired," "stressed," and "bored." LGBTQ students reported the greatest anxiety and depression and least positive feelings such as acceptance and psychological safety.[9]

Of course, teaching is stressful; we care about our students. They all have unique needs. We're wondering how best to support them. We're going to their performances and keeping a full schedule and trying to be humans with responsibilities to ourselves and our loved ones outside of teaching. But just like we learned in regard to nervous system function, stress is a natural biological response that is supposed to end so that systems can return to balance. As polyvagal researcher and educator Deb Dana writes in *Anchored*, "The ability to flexibly move between stages is a sign of wellbeing and resilience. It is when we are caught in dysregulation, unable to find our way back to regulation, that we feel distress."[10] There's a reason that I've buried this information eight chapters into our work together, and van Dernoot Lipsky expresses it perfectly:

> When it comes to caring for ourselves while caring for others and our planet, we often choose to believe that, somehow, we are different. Somehow our capabilities must be greater. Somehow we are entitled to a less arduous, less introspective, less involved role in our own well-being. In fact, we are not.[11]

Helping professionals are often the very worst patients; we are constantly assessing and directing others, but we don't apply the things we know to help ourselves.

Signs You May Be Operating beyond Capacity

Becoming trauma-informed is a crucial component of professional practice if we are to provide holistic vocal care to every singer we encounter. But as we begin to study trauma's far-reaching effects, we may start to feel overwhelmed, frustrated, or angry at the way humans can treat one another. We may also experience a renewed sense of purpose, a commitment to change, and an eagerness to engage in our work in new ways. Give yourself permission to put the book down, take a few deep breaths, and get a clear sense of the numerous thoughts and sensations that are arising for you.

We turn our focus now to the steps necessary for *the teacher* to create the steady ground from which to engage deeply with this work. As we move into this discussion, it is valuable to remember that a critical difference between voice teacher training and that of mental health professionals is the requirement to be involved in a therapeutic process throughout the course of study. This component of work helps future therapists learn to hold complexity with less judgment and reactivity and provides the space to learn more about themselves such as habitual responses to stress. What less than ideal behaviors do you fall back on when you are tired or stressed? Trauma awareness helps us to view our working relationships in new ways, but if you start to feel like you're the only one who can help a student or understand them clearly, that's a sign that you may need more supportive structures in place for yourself.

Laura van Dernoot Lipsky is the founder and director of the Trauma Stewardship Institute and author of *Trauma Stewardship: An Everyday Guide to Caring for Self While Caring for Others* and *The Age of Overwhelm*. Widely recognized as a pioneer in the field of trauma exposure, she has worked locally, nationally, and internationally for more than three decades.[12]

In *Trauma Stewardship*, van Dernoot Lipsky has provided an essential resource for professionals who contact trauma on a regular basis. While the book's primary audience is social workers, environmental activists, and healers and advocates on the front lines of traumatic experience, voice professionals may find solace and renewed purpose knowing that being affected by our work is not a weakness or a liability. As you begin to explore what trauma-informed care looks like in your professional setting, I recommend jotting down the following sixteen items. They are common signs of trauma exposure response, explained in great detail in *Trauma Stewardship*. If you start to experience one or more of the following, slow down, read the entirety of *Trauma Stewardship*, and seek some support for yourself.

Sixteen Signs of Trauma Exposure Response*

*For voice professionals, the list below may also provide some warning signs that you are overstepping professional boundaries, becoming enmeshed in your students' pain and experiences, and/or operating beyond your own training, ethical boundaries, and safe limits.[13]

- feeling hopeless and helpless
- a sense that one can never do enough
- hypervigilance
- diminished creativity
- inability to embrace complexity
- minimizing (as in, "people have it much worse than I do so I should suck it up")
- chronic exhaustion/physical ailments
- inability to listen/deliberate avoidance of people, situations, conversations
- dissociative moments
- sense of persecution
- guilt
- fear
- anger and cynicism

inability to empathize/numbing
addictions
grandiosity (an inflated sense of importance related to one's work)

Paul Griffin, the theater director featured in *The Body Keeps the Score* says, "You cannot fix, help, or save the young people you are working with. What you can do is work side by side with them, help them to understand their vision, and realize it with them. By doing that you give them back control. We're healing trauma without anyone ever mentioning the word."[14]

Just Don't Say "Self-Care"

As we begin to practice more empathy and compassion in our professional practice, we must also turn these qualities back upon ourselves. Van Dernoot Lipsky explains that "[i]f we've laid the groundwork internally to listen to ourselves with empathy, we may be able to hear others' concerns, feedback, and reflections in a more open way as well."[15] As discussed in chapter 7, if we view ourselves with cruelty or disdain, this can't help but leech into our interactions with others. Van Dernoot Lipsky advises that we must develop the capacity to stay present in the face of challenges, maintain an internal sense of sturdiness, and be skilled at maintaining an integrated self.[16] We can only sustain the challenging work we do, and the empathy required, if we remain dedicated to mindfulness and personal insight.[17]

This may sound like a lovely fairy tale to you, or you may be rolling your eyes at yet another book encouraging that most despised and misunderstood of buzzwords: *self-care*. I work deliberately to avoid this term whenever possible because for some it conjures up images of bubble baths and scented candles; for others, a glass (or bottle) of wine. Because so many of us consider this concept from a place of burnout, we may imagine destructive behaviors like being rude and disrespectful to people who irritate us, or flagrantly breaking the law. I think it's simple. What kind of person do you want to be in the world? Are your choices and actions getting you closer to that goal, or further away? If you're still not convinced about the concept of self-care, Deb Dana suggests considering this topic in response to your nervous system states.[18]

When I am in dorsal collapse and disconnection, I feel _____ and self-care looks like _____.

When I am in a state of sympathetic mobilization, I feel _____ and self-care looks like _____.

When I'm anchored in a ventral state, I feel _____ and self-care looks like _____.

It's not useful to bully yourself into being social if you are in a state of dorsal shut down. In fact, in some states, self-care might not be possible at all. In those instances, the best care you can offer yourself might be going to bed and starting over tomorrow. In some sympathetic states, you may feel energized and sociable (I often want to go out with friends after a performance ends). However, when I'm in a sympathetic state that approaches panic, I need to walk by myself or have a soft conversation with a trusted friend so that I can make eye contact and remember that I have a physical body and I won't feel this way forever. Dana also suggests thinking of self-care in four areas: spiritual, mental, relational, physical.[19] Different states need different things, and it's best to develop your library when you are feeling relatively settled and at ease.

Clear It Out

As Lynn Eustis discusses in *The Teacher's Ego*, every singing teacher is responsible for making peace with their personal musical history. Admittedly, this can be extraordinarily painful, but holding onto these wounds is another example of Menakem's "dirty pain." The classical voice world has been just as damaging to us as it can be to our students. We have dealt with countless rejections, we've encountered abusive training, and we might just feel angry that we've developed immense skill but were never anointed as the "Next Big Thing" by a mercurial and outdated system. You are a singer, you deserve to sing, and you deserve for singing to be something that adds joy to your life. Van Dernoot Lipsky offers guiding questions for your self-inquiry: "I encourage you to ask yourself if what you are doing in your life is working for you on all levels of your being. Does it edify you? Do you use it to escape your life? Does it bring you joy? Does it support your ego?"[20] I started to ask similar questions about singers a few years ago, after encountering many of the same singers in a decade of performing throughout New England, but I've since noticed that it's the same everywhere I go. If you have come to hate singing and it hurts you so badly, why do you continue doing it? You have a choice. You always have the option of reclaiming your voice, and using it however you want, gatekeepers be damned. Is singing Tosca at La Scala really the only way you can feel that your efforts have been meaningful? Where did that dream begin, and is it even yours? The bottom line is that miserable teachers should not teach, and miserable singers should not sing. Life is too short. You deserve better, and the part that may burn going down is, so do your students and your audiences.

Further questions for inquiry from *Trauma Stewardship*:[21]

> Why am I doing what I am doing?
> Is this working for me?
> Where am I putting my focus?
> What is my plan B?

After you have taken some time to reflect on what you've been through and where you are now, Resmaa Menakem offers an amazing blueprint for what he calls a "gratifying growth routine."[22] Combined, these elements help us maintain our minds, spirits, and physical bodies to increase our resilience. Menakem recommends the following:

- Enough sleep
- Good nutrition
- Enough water
- Regular exercise (at least thirty minutes a day, five days a week) because it can "increase your resilience, strengthen your heart, improve your mood, release endorphins and other feel-good chemicals, reduce tension, and support your overall physical and mental health."
- Do one small, simple thing every day that feels good
- Some form of meditation, prayer, or chanting. (This sentiment is echoed by Laura van Dernoot Lipsky in *Trauma Stewardship*. She adds that "a daily centering practice is not just a healthy option; it is our best hope of creating a truly sustainable life for ourselves.")[23]

Van Dernoot Lipsky adds that all helping professionals need a network of support: peers or people outside your profession who can listen deeply, understand your passion for your work, and reflect back to you when you may be displaying warning signs of distress.[24] This may sound like a lot of work, but Menakem reminds us that we can move incrementally and add subtle changes in routine over time. These practices prepare us to face daily challenges with clarity and less reactivity. We bolster our sense of internal steadiness, which helps us to hold complexity with more ease. "In the process, you also grow, create more room in your nervous system for flow and coherence, and build your capacity for further growth."[25] Committing to these practices represents another form of clean pain.

> Clean pain is about choosing integrity over fear. It is about letting go of what is familiar but harmful, finding the best parts of yourself, and making a leap—with no guarantee of safety or praise. This healing does not happen in your head. It

happens in your body. And it is more likely to happen in a body that can stay settled in the midst of conflict and uncertainty.

The alternative paths of avoidance, blame and denial are paved with dirty pain. When people respond from their most wounded parts and choose dirty pain, they only create more of it, both for themselves and for other people.[26]

After all, the expressive art of singing is about telling the truth about the human condition and conveying your truest self to an audience. Bessel van der Kolk reminds us that "this requires pushing through blockages to discover your own truth, exploring and examining your own internal experience so that it can emerge in your voice and body on stage."[27] If any of us desire to teach communicative performance to anyone in any medium, we must undertake this journey for ourselves.

Creating a Trauma-Informed Culture

Ideally, you won't be alone in your desire to transform your practice and the ways that we support students. Some healthcare entities are already looking for ways to foster a culture of staff wellness, a critical element in developing a trauma-informed approach. The Center for Health Care Strategies has created resources[28] to help organizations transform to better facilitate the care of individuals with trauma. These guidelines acknowledge that it's essential for employees to take the time to care for themselves so that they can provide the best care possible. The guidelines also recognize that

> [s]taff members may also come to this work with their own histories of trauma. Organizations without safeguards in place to allow staff to safely process their emotions may be exposing employees to secondary traumatic stress, vicarious trauma, and burnout, all of which may inhibit their ability to provide high-quality care and may increase staff turnover.

Other strategies include a flexible policy around paid time off and making it clear that mental health days are just as real as traditional "sick days," reinforcing the value that emotional and mental well-being are critical for job performance. The guidelines also advocate for subtle shifts like making sure that you eat lunch somewhere other than your desk, including short breaks for movement throughout the day, and adding a few minutes before each shift for a meditation to help clear the mind and make staff more receptive to whatever will come their way.

Secure Attachment Skills

> Bowlby saw attachment as the secure base from which a child moves out into the world. Over the subsequent five decades, research has firmly established that having a safe haven promotes self-reliance and instills a sense of sympathy and helpfulness to others in distress.[29]

In chapter 3, we briefly discussed secure attachment and its benefits, but we mostly focused on attachment adaptations and how to recognize them in students and ourselves. Now we'll discuss steps that teachers can take to help build secure attachment in their relationships with students and in their personal lives. Poole Heller explains that secure attachment is actually our default wiring, and even if you didn't grow up with secure attachment, you can learn it.[30] When we grow into secure attachment, we feel protected and cared for, we know that we have compassionate caregivers who are on our side, and we develop a sense of autonomy and independence. We become more aware of our own thoughts, feelings, and reactions. We regulate our nervous system more easily and we grow more resilient. We are free to make our own discoveries and mistakes, and then to reconnect with caregivers and remember their loving support.[31] Bessel van der Kolk explains that "[a] secure attachment combined with the cultivation of competency builds an *internal locus of control*, the key factor in healthy coping throughout life."[32] When someone has developed secure attachment skills, either from their family of origin or as part of ongoing healing work in adulthood, they learn what makes them feel good and bad, and perhaps what every voice teacher hopes for their students: they develop a sense of agency, and an awareness that their actions can change how they feel. As we've been discussing the difference between difficult things and traumatic circumstances, secure attachment skills can play a role in helping singers to see the difference. Van der Kolk says, "Securely attached kids learn the difference between situations they can control and situations where they need help. They learn that they can play an active role when faced with difficult situations." This is how voice teachers can ethically prepare singers for life as artists. It's not coddling. We can practice secure attachment skills in the studio, which help students develop their own sense of agency, and which helps teachers to cultivate healthy support in their own lives. This is crucial to voice work because people need to feel safe and held before they are going to go deeper with their explorations of breath and body, risk taking, habit change, and expressive communication. When we experience secure attachment, we're able to let our guard down and fully be ourselves, which is critical for artistic exploration. In van der Kolk's words, when we learn secure attachment, we "have a lifetime advantage—a kind of buffer against the worst that fate can hand [us]."[33]

In *The Power of Attachment*, Poole Heller lays out secure attachment skills that can be summed up for voice practitioners as follows:[34]

- Work hard to be emotionally present during sessions. Put your own emotional stuff aside to the best of your ability so you can listen clearly and without reactivity.
- Listen deeply to your clients and make space for them to ask questions.
- Do your best to notice their emotional state when they enter the room. If someone seems very down or lost in their own thoughts, coming at them with a lot of energy may be disorienting. It's best to meet them where they are and let them feel what they're feeling. As you attune to them, their nervous system will begin to settle as they understand that they are being seen and matched.

Developmental psychiatrist Ed Tronick has been studying social emotional development in infants since the 1970s. His research shows that when we are in sync with a caregiver, our sense of connection is reflected in a steady heartbeat and breath rate, as well as a low level of stress hormones. "[our] body is calm; so are [our] emotions."[35]

Talk to Them

One of the ways that we can cultivate a climate of care is by taking time to truly get to know our students. I do an initial "intake session" at the beginning of my work with a student so that I can learn a bit about their musical history, level of training, and anything else they would like to share with me that might affect our work together. Admittedly, this sometimes catches students off guard, and they aren't sure what to say in that first meeting. But it conveys that who they are matters to me and to our work. They will frequently circle back and say, "Something I should have mentioned . . . " and this is a wonderful sign that they understand that what they share will be valued.

This also means that teachers must be brave enough to talk to students about what is hard in their learning process. Are they hung up on a rhythmic error that they can't correct? Are they singing an interval incorrectly? These are clear, fact-based issues that are easily solved with some focused teaching. Many of my students are successful musicians because they have great ears, and their musical literacy lags behind their recall and mimicking skills. They may have a hard time teaching themselves repertoire at the piano because they can't play it yet, and they may rely heavily on available recordings and the miracle of YouTube. If this is the case, I acknowledge this truth, and also explain how we are hoping to bolster the student's skills throughout their degree program with musicianship classes and piano instruction. But until those skills catch up, I talk about how recordings can be useful in the learning process, and when we need to let them go and focus on our own work. I can't yell at them for not having better skills, because that's what they're in school to learn. If they could be functional professionals with such a limited skill set, I would encourage them to go out there and get to work! But the truth is, if they're in school, some part of them has acknowledged that the skills they have so far are not enough to help them reach their personal and professional goals. If I explain how the curriculum supports those goals, and I also support the student while they are building those skills, they can cultivate a sense of pride in the choice to attend school, and perhaps a tiny extra bit of motivation to get up for those 8 a.m. classes and do that harmonic analysis.

Listen

We can't just begin a lesson with a chit-chat about the weather or how hard it is to find a parking space and expect that this will foster growth. We need to deeply listen to what our students share with us and work to keep it in mind as skill development occurs. If they get frustrated in a lesson and mention that something is hard for them, ask, "Why do you think that is?" and be present to whatever it is the student is able to notice. Just as we are asking the students to cultivate nonjudgmental awareness of their thoughts and habits, so must we as teachers begin to accept their responses as accurate representations of what they're thinking and feeling in the moment. We need to lead students gently through this. The teacher might be able to see that some emotional block is holding a student back, but it's not up to us to diagnose or interfere with that very personal process. Sometimes I will indicate to a student that if they are stuck in some way that there may be "something going on in there that I don't have access to." This lets the student see how something internal is restricting their progress and gives them the option of deciding whether/when/how to proceed with investigating. In the moment, students will often let that comment land and then continue with whatever it was they were doing. Sometimes weeks (or even semesters) later, they mention that they're seeing a therapist, or casually say that they've made progress on a big issue that has seemed to make singing easier. In this way, I point the student toward something and let *them* figure out what to do with that information. Sometimes it's nothing. I don't insert myself into their healing process. As therapist Lori Gottleib writes in *Maybe You Should Talk to Someone*,

> Rather than steering people straight to the heart of the problem, we nudge them to arrive there on their own, because the most powerful truths—the ones people take most seriously—are those they come to, little by little, on their own. . . . [S]ome discomfort is unavoidable for the process to be effective.[36]

I had a student who spent many of their lessons unloading about the difficulties they were experiencing in other classes, with their roommates, socially, you name it. I often felt like they were not really seeking advice, just a sympathetic listener. This is where I first started practicing phrases like "That sounds really hard," or "I remember that feeling," that displayed empathy, but I didn't try to jump into the situation to become the hero or rescuer. My fixing impulse is quite overdeveloped, so it took a lot for me to get into a patient headspace and remind myself that I couldn't solve this student's problems. After several weeks of this, I tried as kindly as I could to say something along the lines of "I'm happy to listen to you and I'm glad that you feel safe enough to tell me what's going on. I do wonder sometimes if you're getting enough information about your singing." In this way, I was able to validate that they needed someone to talk to. I was also able to drop a hint that I could probably be more effective in their life by using our lesson time for more vocal instruction, but they were able to process that on their own time and decide how to move forward. What happened next is the kind of thing that people write novels or make movies about: after the summer, this student returned utterly transformed. They had begun meditating; they had done some deep healing work that had nothing to do with me. They were calmer, focused, and they worked really hard in the remainder of their time at school and by all accounts have a really beautiful life. I didn't have to bully them into changing or give them a lecture about "wasting time." The work we needed to do first was give them a space to learn how they were feeling. Then they noticed that they were really unhappy, and *they* did something about it.

Ultimately, boundaries are created and defined by you. We can't control the behavior of others, but we can choose how we will respond to certain types of communication. For example, my students know that they can email me at any time, but I stop checking my school email at 9:00 p.m. My cell phone is only for last-minute messages, like when someone is running late or has suddenly become sick. If a new student sends me a text message outside of these parameters, I will discuss my boundary with them when we next meet. Sometimes difficult conversations arise. Again, we can't control the reaction of a colleague or student, but we can clearly state, "I understand that you are upset but if you continue to yell at me or use derogatory language, I will choose to end this conversation and regroup at a future time." Admittedly, some students have a lot of situations or language that can cause a high level of activation. We'll never be able to anticipate what might be activating for someone else, but if you as an educator are modeling boundaries well, your students will also see how one can hold a protective line around others. The goal is not to get the world to walk on eggshells around you; unfortunately, that's never going to happen. Your responsibility is to treat yourself with honesty and gentleness and find ways to be productive and get your work done, even knowing that things will always be going wrong.

Attend to Ruptures

Teachers also need to be mindful of the need for relationship repair.[37] We're human, and sometimes things go wrong. For example, I had a student who was really struggling with their anxiety. They had a hard time making it to lessons and staying on top of learning lesson material. We had been building a good rapport, and I was happy about their progress, but (similar to the student above) I was getting nervous that we were spending too much lesson time talking and not enough time on skill building. In the next lesson, I decided that my agenda was to work harder to keep them on task and not let them distract me. I asked them to do something, and they made a legitimate discovery and connected what they had just experienced with something else in their life. Ordinarily, this is one of my favorite things in the studio; students make such interesting connections, and this imbues their work with meaning in a way that I could never manufacture. But that day, I cut them off and I told them that I didn't need to know about it. They turned red and looked as though I had slapped them across the face. I felt as sick and sad as if I had, indeed, slapped them. After the lesson ended, I felt as though months of trust building had been thrown out the window, all because I had decided that my agenda was more important than my student. After I had a chance to process my feelings, I sent an email to apologize, and I set about regaining their trust.

If the breach happens the other way, and a student acts inappropriately, or fails to meet established standards or guidelines, try to be open to any effort they make toward repair, even if it's not exactly what you want or would expect of a more developed adult with more complex emotional skills. It's up to us to recognize singers' humanity and the imperfect journey toward growth.

If the Teacher Has Avoidant Attachment

If the teacher is the one in the studio who has developed an avoidant attachment adaptation, they may be unsympathetic and unresponsive to student needs. We see this frequently when teachers say, "Well, no one taught me to . . . " Many academic institutions are home to grudge-bearing gatekeepers (think: "*I* had to suffer in this particular way, so you do too"). Because avoidant folks have difficulty recognizing their own needs, it is very difficult to view even the most basic human needs proportionately. They may habitually identify their students as "weak" or "soft" or "too sensitive." Teachers can grow in this area by practicing secure attachment skills (see above), learning more about mental health in students, and examining their attachment history.

If the Teacher Has Ambivalent Attachment

The most difficult challenge for the teacher with anxious attachment is the conclusion of the relationship with each student. In essence, all of our students leave us, either because they have finished their course of study, or because they've changed their major, or decided to work with another teacher. The latter can feel especially painful, as though you've done something wrong, or you have failed the student. Keep in mind that our work is in support of the *student's* needs. As you continue to understand your own attachment patterns, you may find more ease around such situations. Unfortunately, many of us work with young or developing adults, who mostly don't understand the nuances of professional dialogue and asking for what they want in a clear way. Most of the time, the student will unintentionally hurt you before they muster the courage to ask to leave the studio. They may be very vocal about their discomfort among their peers (or *your* peers), and this can trigger insecurity and doubt in the teacher. It will be very important for you to process your own feelings about the situation among *your* support network; it's not appropriate to end up in a break-up type argument with a student. Even if you think the student is making a mistake, it is the mark of a true professional to educate the student about how they could handle such matters with more tact in the future and then to genuinely wish them well.

Notes

1. Laura van Dernoot Lipsky, Connie Burk, and Jon R. Conte, *Trauma Stewardship: An Everyday Guide to Caring for Self While Caring for Others*, first ed. (Oakland, CA: Berrett-Koehler, 2009), 12.
2. Rupa Marya and Raj Patel, *Inflamed: Deep Medicine and the Anatomy of Injustice*, first ed. (New York: Farrar Straus and Giroux, 2021), 91.
3. Julietta A. Sheng, Natalie J. Bales, Sage A. Myers, Anna I. Bautista, Mina Roueinfar, Taben M. Hale, and Robert J. Handa, "The Hypothalamic-Pituitary-Adrenal Axis: Development, Programming Actions of Hormones, and Maternal-Fetal Interactions, Frontiers in Behavioral Neuroscience 14 (2020): https://www.frontiersin.org/articles/10.3389/fnbeh.2020.601939/full#:~:text=A%20major%20component%20of%20the,autonomic%20nervous%20system%20(ANS).

4. Marya and Patel, *Inflamed*, 91.
5. Ibid., 92.
6. Ibid., 284.
7. Marc A. Brackett, *Permission to Feel: Unlocking the Power of Emotions to Help Our Kids Ourselves and Our Society Thrive*, first ed. (New York: Celadon Books, 2019), 3.
8. Lipsky, *Trauma Stewardship* 3.
9. Brackett, *Permission to Feel* 191.
10. Deb Dana, *Anchored: How to Befriend Your Nervous System Using Polyvagal Theory* (Boulder, CO: Sounds True, 2021), 22.
11. Lipsky et al., *Trauma Stewardship*, 123.
12. "Laura van Dernoot Lipsky," The Trauma Stewardship Institute, https://traumastewardship.com/laura-van-dernoot-lipsky/.
13. Lipsky et al., *Trauma Stewardship*, 47–113.
14. Bessel A. Van der Kolk, *The Body Keeps the Score: Brain Mind and Body in the Healing of Trauma* (New York: Penguin Books, 2015), 344.
15. Lipsky et al., *Trauma Stewardship*, 15.
16. Ibid., 18.
17. Ibid., 21.
18. Dana, *Anchored*, 153.
19. Ibid., 155.
20. Lipsky et al., *Trauma Stewardship*, 120.
21. Ibid., 147–83.
22. Resmaa Menakem, *My Grandmother's Hands: Racialized Trauma and the Pathway to Mending Our Hearts and Bodies* (Las Vegas: Central Recovery Press, 2017), 161.
23. Lipsky et al., *Trauma Stewardship*, 230.
24. Ibid., 184.
25. Menakem, *My Grandmother's Hands*, 165.
26. Ibid., 166.
27. Van der Kolk, *The Body Keeps the Score*, 337.
28. Meryl Schulman and Christopher Menschner, "Laying the Groundwork for Trauma-Informed Care," January 2018, https://www.traumainformedcare.chcs.org/wp-content/uploads/Brief-Laying-the-Groundwork-for-TIC_11.10.20.pdf.
29. Van der Kolk, *The Body Keeps the Score*, 113.
30. Diane Poole Heller, *The Power of Attachment: How to Create Deep and Lasting Intimate Relationships* (Boulder, CO: Sounds True, 2019), 19.
31. Ibid., 27–32.
32. Van der Kolk, *The Body Keeps the Score*, 115.
33. Ibid., 112.
34. Poole Heller, *The Power of Attachment*, 33–51.
35. Van der Kolk, *The Body Keeps the Score*, 114.
36. Lori Gottlieb, *Maybe You Should Talk to Someone: A Therapist, Her Therapist, and Our Lives Revealed* (Boston: Houghton Mifflin Harcourt, 2019), 124.
37. Poole Heller, *The Power of Attachment*, 44.

9

Practical Tools and Best Practices

Emily Jaworski Koriath and Lauren A. Cook

Heather McCornack offers her perspective on trauma-informed voice care:

> I began studying trauma informed voice care after I started teaching yoga for people in trauma recovery and eating disorder recovery. A 2017 study published in the journal *Eating and Weight Disorders* reported that almost one third of the musicians studied were currently experiencing or had at one time suffered from an eating disorder.[1] This means acknowledging that specific obstacles stood between some of my students and their ability to sing freely and with creative ease.
>
> Education and my own lived experience have taught me that the concept of embodiment feels largely inaccessible when you don't feel safe within your own body. A full breath is often out of reach due to increased tension in the abdominal muscles and the reluctance to experience this sense of body expansion. There is likely increased tension in the abdominal muscles, laryngeal muscles, areas in the neck and shoulders. They may also be experiencing hormonal imbalances and other physical side effects that affect the voice. All of these contribute to inefficient, strained singing and are symptoms of which to be aware. Voice students with or healing eating disorders are also living with an enormous amount of emotional stress and pain. Offering therapeutic advice is outside a voice instructor's scope of practice but we can be ready to suggest professional resources should a student request them.
>
> Trauma informed voice care provides me with tools to reach these students with sensitivity. It is an opportunity to offer support in a unique way and show students how singing could be a way back into their body. I start by shifting my teaching language away from expectation, striving, or judgment, and toward curiosity, compassion, and grace. "I wonder what would happen if . . . ," "It

sounds like today has been hard. Let's start with gentle humming . . . ," "I love how you were aware of what you needed today . . . " I adjust repertoire requirements, performance expectations, lesson duration or frequency for a while as I let the student take the lead. Empowering them with choice helps a student notice what feels right and good to them in that moment. Honoring their choice is a trauma sensitive tool that not only builds trust between teacher and singer but also empowers a singer to trust their own inner-knowing.

I take a gentle approach with the breath. Singers expect a lot from their breath, and it can be a source of frustration. I want the breath to feel like a quiet invitation to discover sensation. "Let's start today by feeling your breath come in and out your nose. Notice the pace of your breath without feeling the need to change anything," "Take a breath in and then exhale fully. Do you think your exhale is longer than your inhale? What would that be like?," "As you inhale, what do you notice in your body? Does your attention land somewhere specific? Do you feel any kind of movement?" With time and practice, the breath becomes more familiar and resiliency begins to increase. I might then start to introduce more robust breath practices.

When it comes to vocal warm-ups, I focus on freedom and sounding versus precision and control. I applaud mistakes and inaccuracy, acknowledging the bravery in risk as opposed to the limitations of perfection. Warm-ups can be an opportunity to invite some levity into the voice lesson, which almost always supports a spirit of curiosity. When it comes to choosing repertoire, I lessen the degree of musical difficulty and focus on student preference and artistic expression. Some days, I might not address technique at all. If the student is engaged and connected to the music and their voice, I do not want to disrupt that moment to give feedback that probably feels like criticism. This is a glorious opportunity for the singer to practice embodiment. When you spend a lot of time on the outside, it can be hard to think of reasons to go back in, but singing can be a remembering of that goodness. After they finish, I ask them to give me feedback based on sensation, not sound. "Can you remember where you felt that sustained note in your body?," "Remember how we practiced a long exhale at the beginning of your lesson? Did you notice a place in the song where you also felt that?," "How did it feel to sing the lyrics in this section?" Eating disorder recovery is a very long process. I have seen trauma-informed voice care transform singing into a powerful recovery tool. It is a way to share someone's authentic voice and explore their unique artistry. Providing a space for those discoveries has not only helped my students but transformed the lens through which I teach.

Heather McCornack
MM Voice Performance, Kansas State University
RYT 300, trauma-informed yoga teacher, teaching faculty at Yoga for Eating Disorders

Two Existing Musical Frameworks: Social Emotional Learning and Trauma-Informed Choral Pedagogy

Having read this far and after being presented with so much information, it's only logical that some voice teachers may be feeling overwhelmed about the practicalities of implementing the principles of trauma-informed care into their work. A close look into the wider field of music education research demonstrates that voice professionals are not the only ones being asked to consider a broader view of their students' humanity. Though impossible to capture adequately in a few brief paragraphs, existing scholarship on both social–emotional learning in the music classroom and trauma-informed choral pedagogy hint at best practices that are easily adapted into voice work.

Social–Emotional Learning

Teachers who have had experience in the American public school system may already be familiar with social–emotional learning (SEL). According to the Collaborative for Academic, Social, and Emotional Learning (CASEL), programs aimed at "educating the whole child" began in Connecticut as early as 1968, though it took almost thirty more years for the term SEL to take hold and for CASEL to be formed. In a 2022 survey, CASEL found that 76 percent of principals and 53 percent of teachers reported that their school used a social–emotional learning system or curricular materials in the 2021–2022 school year.[2] As summarized by CASEL, "SEL is the process through which all young people and adults acquire and apply the knowledge, skills, and attitudes to develop healthy identities, manage emotions and achieve personal and collective goals, feel and show empathy for others, establish and maintain supportive relationships, and make responsible and caring decisions." Luckily for vocal professionals, music educator Scott N. Edgar created *Music Education and Social–Emotional Learning: The Heart of Teaching Music* in 2017.[3] In the book, Edgar acknowledges that music educators are not trained as counselors and often feel unprepared to address SEL topics in the classroom. Perhaps the applied studio is the easiest place to begin implementing these elements due to the personal nature of our interactions with students and the emotional requirements of effective vocal performance.

SEL consists of five key components, listed here with explanations by Edgar:

- Self-awareness, including "recognizing emotions; accurate self-perception; acknowledging strengths, needs, and values; self-efficacy; and spirituality."

- Social awareness, which "includes perspective, empathy, appreciating diversity, and respect."
- Responsible decision making, which includes "identifying problems, problem solving, and personal responsibility. Identifying and developing appropriate responses in difficult situations."
- Self-management, which focuses on "impulse control, stress management, self-motivation, discipline, goal-setting, and organizational skills"; and
- Relationship skills, or "communication, social engagement, building and maintaining relationships, working cooperatively, negotiating refusal, and conflict management."[4]

Many of these principles are *already at work* in our interactions in the studio: recognizing emotions, acknowledging strengths and needs, perspective and empathy, problem solving, self-motivation, discipline, goal-setting, communication, and working cooperatively are all part of a set of skills required of all vocal students. While geared toward the American K–12 school system, curriculum guides and tools are available through CASEL, the Yale Center for Emotional Intelligence, and other SEL organizations, and can provide how-to guides for educators on discussing these topics more directly with students. The pillars above represent a learnable set of skills; if a student seems to lack clarity or experience with a particular skill, it is imperative for the teacher to remember that this is most likely due to an incomplete understanding, meaning that it's something that can be improved with time and attention.

Edgar also highlights five tools to help teachers support students while maintaining their own ethical and personal boundaries. As we discuss SEL skills with students, it is likely that they may begin to confide in us about the development of these skills, presence or absence of them in their care environment or family of origin, and challenges they may be facing while learning to implement the skills. Edgar diligently reiterates throughout the text that music educators are not counselors; but in order to stay present to our students' needs and minimize the risk of re-traumatization, he stressed that the music teacher's responsibilities in difficult conversations are listening to the student actively, without preparing a response or centering our own feelings; questioning the student with open-ended questions that help *the student* gain clarity around their thoughts and feelings; reframing the situation together; and empathizing with the student or acknowledging the difficulty they're experiencing and the skills required to move beyond the challenge.[5] I'll use a recent experience in the studio to illustrate some of these skills in action.

A student arrived at their lesson looking visibly shaken: staring into space and on the verge of tears. I started the conversation the way I always do when I start a lesson.

Teacher: How are you?

Student: Not okay, if I'm being honest. Can I sit down?

Teacher: Of course, you can. Is there anything I can do to help?

Student: [describes an activating event that came up during an acting exercise in class] ... and it brought up this really horrible thing that happened, and now I can't stop thinking about it.

Teacher: Wow. I'm so sorry that you are feeling so rattled by this.

Student: Honestly it feels better just being able to talk about it.

Teacher: I am really happy to hear that. Do you want a few minutes to just hang out with the feeling-better feeling?

Student: Yeah, that sounds really good. [student takes a deep breath]. I'm sorry for dumping all this on you. I know that's not what voice lessons are for.

Teacher: You don't have to apologize for anything. Could you have sung the way that you felt when you walked into the room?

Student: (laughs)

Teacher: Sometimes we just need to put down the things we are carrying before we can get back to work.

Yes, this really happened. If you read closely, you might notice that at no time did I offer the student advice or offer to fix their problem. I listened carefully to what they had to say, empathized by stressing that this was a very hard situation for them, and just got them to slow down and to see the issue with a little more spaciousness. It's easy for people to feel overwhelmed by what they're experiencing, to the point that they almost don't perceive anything else in the world around them. By giving the student a chance to express what was on their mind, and by avoiding the natural inclination to move in and become the fixer, *the student* was able to viscerally feel that they were not powerless in the situation, that their reaction to stress was understandable and natural, and that I would not run away or judge them harshly for having intense feelings. I demonstrated that I will be there, I am capable of listening, and that whatever the student shares with me will not diminish my respect for them or my belief in their ability.

Trauma-Informed Choral Pedagogy

In addition to the aforementioned *Queering Vocal Pedagogy*, William Sauerland also penned a recent article in the *Choral Journal*, published by the American Choral Directors' Association (ACDA), explaining the principles of trauma-informed care (discussed in chapter 6) and applying them to choral pedagogy. Sauerland begins by reiterating that trauma-informed pedagogy (TIP) is not only helpful in teaching students with a history of trauma, but it also benefits all students as teachers work to reduce possible stressors in the classroom and minimize potentially activating behaviors and scenarios. In the article's preface, Sauerland provides four brief vignettes of common rehearsal elements, viewed through a trauma-informed lens. These everyday occurrences—slamming a door, starting a "massage train" as part of vocal warm-ups, enforcing gender stereotypes through performance attire, and scheduling additional rehearsals without notice—look different through the lens of trauma-informed pedagogy.[6] Sauerland reminds readers that it would be impossible to remove all possible trauma triggers from a classroom environment (or any environment), but as we adopt the principles of trauma-informed care we can "bolster the safety and well-being" of the singers in our care. Trauma-informed care does not seek to heal a student's trauma but serves to help educators understand *how* trauma might play a role in students' lives. As Sauerland explains,

> Although music has the power to positively support the well-being of singers, selecting repertoire to help "heal" a singer is beyond the bounds of TIP. Like trauma-informed care, TIP is a model for compassion and care, not a directive to use choir as a place of healing. Though the therapeutic and restorative capacity of music may guide singers to improved wellness, trauma-related health issues should be treated by a mental health professional. The potential for music to ease suffering is immeasurable, but it is beyond the boundary of most choir directors, unless trained and serving as a music therapist, to treat posttraumatic stress.

Tools for Working with Attachment Adaptations

How Can We Work with Avoidant Attachment?

Because of the instinct to avoid emotion, singers with avoidant attachment can default to the factual, logical, and analytical, and display a bias toward action. These folks will often just want to be told what to do. If you suspect a student is presenting with avoidant attachment, try being more concise in your verbal instructions, because the singer is likely to get lost in the details or become overwhelmed by what they consider excessive words.[7] An impulse toward creative expression may not be a high priority to the student with avoidant attachment, and if they are encouraged to "be expressive" before they know how, they may copy others' gestures, or overlay movement in a scripted fashion in an attempt to "do it right." Avoidant folks will also present with a tendency toward gesture inhibition and an overall lack of body connection and awareness.[8] This is yet another reason that it's important to let singers discover a range of expressive gestures on their own terms and in their own time. One of my favorite directives from the studio of Dr. Eustis is to "stand still and tell the truth." I pass this on to my students all the time, as a way of reminding them that it's actually *important* that their interpretation of a song is different from anyone else's and should come from their authentic humanity. I wouldn't necessarily assign this student a flashy character number right off the bat, though we might work ourselves toward that after a few semesters together. I don't believe that we can force people beyond their personalities with daring repertoire choices. The most successful approach will be slow and systematic. This student will need you to use studio time to develop procedures for analyzing texts; you might have the student boil each phrase down to a modern, easy-to-understand equivalent, or to a prominent emotional state. They are capable of great artistry but will need tools and structure to get there (see figures 9.1, 9.2, and 9.3).

Studio Adaptations to Consider

As with all great adaptations, these suggestions are specifically geared to support students with avoidant attachment but would probably benefit a majority of students. Consider making a habit of asking, "What questions do you have?" to encourage student engagement with the learning process and reinforce the concept that asking questions or needing help is safe.

Provide practice templates for beginning students so your expectations are clear. Figures 9.1 and 9.2 are the templates I created in the height of the COVID-19 pandemic when students were struggling to stay engaged with school.

FIGURE 9.1
Text Analysis Template

Song text in original language	English translation	What this really means
Caro mio ben	dear my beloved	oh sweet person
Credimi almen	believe me at least	please listen
Senza di te	etc.	etc.

> **Figure 9.2. Weekly Practice Log**
>
> 1. Invite your body to the work. Shake out your shoulders. Ask your head to bobble on your spine. Remind yourself where your lungs are. Take a few deep breaths.
> 2. Start with the standard vocal warmup (this is a protocol they all know)
> 3. The skill-building exercises Dr. K asked me to work on are:
> 4. My repertoire focus this week is (no more than two):
> 5. The SPECIFIC issue I am working on is (no more than three! Use measure numbers if applicable!):

I also highly recommend distributing the Mood Map, developed by Marc Brackett and the team at the Yale Center for Emotional Intelligence.[9] The Mood Map is printed on the inside cover of Brackett's book *Permission to Feel*, and the associated app can be found at moodmeterapp.com. The Mood Map was created to help students develop a more nuanced emotional vocabulary; it divides emotions on axes indicating energy and pleasantness. These areas are color-coded into four quadrants. You can ask students to identify the specific emotion of a lyric based on this tool. When I gave this tool to my undergraduate students, a few of them took it upon themselves to download the associated app and begin tracking their daily emotions. I leave a copy on my piano for our discussions on text interpretation.

How Do We Work with Ambivalent Attachment?

A student demonstrating ambivalent/anxious attachment will benefit greatly from your reassurance. The nature of your regular contact with the student through weekly sessions will create a stabilizing influence. This singer may present with hypersensitivity or seem to need a lot of attention from you in the form of emails or surprise visits to your office. In the past, I have wanted to remain cool and aloof with these types of students because I was afraid of them growing dependent on me for something I didn't feel I could reliably provide. As we learned in our discussion of secure attachment skills in chapter 8, the opposite is true: by providing reassurance and consistent presence for our clients, they can learn to stabilize and grow independent.

Studio Adaptations to Consider: Closing Rituals

People who have developed an anxious attachment style are particularly susceptible to what is known as "departure stress," the anxiety that flares in us when someone leaves, even at the natural conclusion of a meeting or class.[10] These students may begin to mistrust your relationship when they are not in your presence. It can be useful to develop a closing routine to end the lesson mutually, and to remind the student what types of support are available even if there is no additional studio time scheduled. This can be difficult when lessons are scheduled back-to-back but taking those last few moments to review what you've covered together, review practice strategies, and remind the student of appropriate ways to be in contact with you if they need additional support between sessions can reassure them of your continued presence.

How Do We Work with Disorganized Attachment?

A singer with a disorganized attachment style may default to freeze as an extreme response to fear. It might look like they are cool or unaffected, but inside, they are feeling the equivalent of the brake and gas pedals of a car being slammed simultaneously. They are producing tremendous energy to survive what's happening, while also suppressing those reactions in the name of safety. Assume the best if you have a student who presents as very detached or aloof, since there may be much bigger things at work. Acknowledge that what they are doing takes courage and may activate some fear patterning in their body, because it activates fear in *any* body. While it's true that you can attempt to force a shift in energy by doing very directed breathing exercises, it gives singers more agency if they can start to explore different nervous system states on their own. Offer a menu of movement: the singer can scan their eyes back and forth (this widens scope of vision and helps verify that no biological threat is actually present); they can wiggle their toes inside their shoes (I conduct my music with my toes, and my students seem to love learning this about me); you could ask a student to stand on their tiptoes and then forcefully drop their heels; or you could ask them to knead their shoulders and arms with their own hands. These strategies can create subtle down-regulation of the nervous system, making it more possible for a student to stay mentally present in the moment.

Studio Adaptations to Consider

With all my students, I openly discuss threat orientation. I acknowledge that most people feel scared about singing in front of others, and we get stuck when we try to ignore or suppress those feelings. They're biologically wired. When I'm feeling silly, I say, "Congratulations! You are primed to survive a bear attack! You are normal!" Rather than fight ourselves, we can minimize these fears by discussing them honestly. I ask students, "Can you describe what feels scary about what you are doing?" or, even more likely, I remind them that our bodies are reacting the exact same way that they would if we saw a bear in school. This makes you biologically *normal*. And then I say that I have never yet seen a bear in school. This creates a moment of levity (or at least eye-rolling) and mitigates potential shame that the student may be feeling about their reactions. Next, we discuss the actual consequences of making mistakes. This is where I remind students that I won't hit them or yell at them, and I won't kick them out of the studio. I remind them that my studio is a place where mistakes are a *celebrated* element of the learning process and that I don't have an alligator hiding under a trap door. This sounds silly, but as social worker and shame researcher Brené Brown says, "shame cannot survive being spoken."[11] When we openly discuss these fears and debunk them, they lose their power.

Incumbent upon you as the teacher, then, is to acknowledge mistakes with clarity and without judgment. Instead of telling my students that they're flat, I say, "Do you hear that the F is under pitch?" One is personal and easy to misinterpret as "I am flat; therefore, I am bad." The latter is an opportunity to reinforce to the student that you are both on the same page. In my studio, the complete conversation goes more like "Do you hear that the F is under pitch? That's because [of a scientific reason] so this is where we [implement a technical concept we have been working on in exercises]."

With all students, we should celebrate things that are going well. Even if the student is not meeting all your standards, work to find *something* to compliment in their work. Perhaps they show up on time every week, or they always have their translation work done. This student might be very musically accurate. Remember that this is a student who is prone to feeling like a failure. They may be most inclined to give up when faced with a challenge. Balance the feedback you're giving them so it's not always pointing out their "flaws."

Teaching Self Compassion

Perhaps one of the most universal elements of learning to acquire any skill is the particularly insidious cruelty we inflict upon ourselves as we do so. I watched one first-year student become red in the face during a lesson, trying incredibly hard to accomplish a specific vocal task. I could tell he was getting intensely upset in a way that seemed disproportionate to the problem at hand. I stopped him so we could talk about this, and so he wouldn't hurt his voice. I asked him, "Pete, would you ever talk to one of your classmates the way that you talk to yourself?" His eyes grew wide with horror, and he covered his open mouth with his hands at the mere thought of inflicting such cruelty on another. Just acknowledging that this is a natural human trait *and that these thoughts are not true, necessary, or helpful*[12] can hopefully help students see this neurological wiring for what it is, and stop being limited by this pattern.

It turns out that the mean voice in our heads has a job, and it's to keep us safe. Kristin Neff has spent her career studying the neuroscience of self-compassion. As Neff explains in *Self-Compassion: The Proven Power of Being Kind to Yourself*, the human species developed based on the strength of our survival skills. Though modern society is more fragmented, we developed in hierarchical social groups; it was safest to stick together as a pack to find food and resources, and to be protected against threat. Straying too far from the group, physically or philosophically, meant increased risk. Making choices that counter the group would have put early humans at greater risk of being outcast, forced to fight for survival alone. While we don't depend as directly on others as we once did, these hard-wired instincts remain.[13]

This biological wiring also comes with a downside, and that's the fact that most often we weaponize it against ourselves. As Neff explains, it's as if we

Figure 9.3. Considering the Audience

Alexander Technique teacher Cathy Madden encourages all performers to include consideration of their audience in their preparation for any piece.[1] The following exercise, adapted from Diane Poole Heller's "protective sphere exercise"[2] can help students learn to somatically track how the perception of an audience affects their body.

As your student sings, ask them to experiment with different positions of their arms. First, have them sing with arms extended out front, hands raised in a gesture that says "stop." Next, try keeping the hands in the same position, but letting the elbows drop so the arms stay closer to the torso. Experiment with turning the palms of the hands upward, having the singer wrap themselves as in a hug, and maybe even widening the arms outward as though preparing the student to receive a hug. After each movement, ask the singer what they notice in the body. As they get closer to their natural physical boundaries, they will begin to feel uncomfortable with some positions. They might notice their pulse quicken, breath become more difficult, or a tightening in the throat. Some of my students just make a weird face or let out a sound of discomfort. This exercise helps the student begin to develop an energetic boundary with an audience. Experimenting with these boundaries helps students to somatically feel their way into a sense of safety; this boundary will look different for everyone.

Notes

1. Cathy Madden, *Integrative Alexander Technique Practice for Performing Artists: Onstage Synergy* (United Kingdom: Intellect Books Limited, 2014).
2. Diane Poole Heller, *The Power of Attachment: How to Create Deep and Lasting Intimate Relationships* (Boulder, CO: Sounds True, 2019), 132.

think that labeling our own flaws and berating ourselves about them shows the group that we are aware of our inadequacies and are working to address them. If we cut ourselves down, we think it will protect us from being rejected by others.[14] Unfortunately, self-criticism is strongly related to depression and dissatisfaction with life.[15] Our students are consistently challenging themselves to push their own boundaries and grow, which in our tribal ancestors would have been seen as threatening. When we take risks of this kind, that evolutionary mechanism for safety and survival kicks into overdrive, so some training about the harmful effects of this internal cruelty will go a long way. Neff reports that one of the most consistent findings in the research is that people who are more self-compassionate tend to be less anxious and depressed.[16] She goes on to explain that our brains have a negativity bias: a strong tendency to notice what's wrong instead of what's right. It makes sense in terms of survival instincts; if you notice that the grass is lying in a different way than it was just a few minutes ago, you might have just detected a predator, and that awareness could save your life. In musician development, training can sometimes focus too heavily on convincing the student of what they are doing wrong. True, we want them to notice when they have made a musical mistake so they can prepare music accurately, and oftentimes the road to technical proficiency begins with noticing when things feel off. But without mindfulness and the ability to notice errors objectively, too often these observations edge down the road of self-cruelty. It's not just that the note is out of tune, it's that *I'm always out of tune; I'll never get it right, but Bethany plays in tune all the time and I'll never be as good as she is; and I should probably quit because I quit everything because I'm a loser*. This thinking process is fueled by fear, shame, and inadequacy.

As every expert on the subject will tell you, we can't consciously suppress emotions.[17] Our goal is not to stop self-criticism from ever arising. Our negativity bias will always be with us, but this doesn't mean that we must believe everything (or anything!) it says. In fact, if we can strip away the cruelty of our inner judge, we may find a lot of useful wisdom. We can use the experience of *being with* what's happening and notice the dialogue taking place. Teachers can model and encourage this in the studio. When a student sings through a piece, an exercise, or a phrase, I like to ask, "What did you like about that?" or "How much of that went according to your plan?" This helps the brain to refocus from "oh, the high note was no good, I took a bad breath, I felt weird the whole time" and the whole automatic litany of self-judgment that seems so easy to tap into. We help our students practice moving through that cloud of doubt to find something constructive. That's a much more helpful place from which to work.

Just like mindfulness, there are studies emerging about the brain science behind self-compassion, something we may be tempted to dismiss as touchy-feely. Studies show that self-compassion relates to less fear, irritability, hostility, and distress,[18] and greater resilience in the face of trauma.[19] Don't we all want those things for our students? If we are hoping to cultivate artists who find joy in the process of discovering and creating, providing them with a biological understanding of the ways their brain circuitry sometimes works against them is an essential part of their training. Neff reports that there is also data supporting the claim that self-compassionate people have better emotional coping skills, as measured by lower cortisol levels and higher heart rate variability, a metric discussed in chapter 1 that is also used as an indicator of coherence among systems of the body. "This suggests that self-compassionate people are able to deal with the challenges life throws their way with greater emotional equanimity."[20]

Lest you fear that self-compassion will make students "soft," be assured that the data suggests the exact opposite. This is because, like we discovered with Carol Dweck's research on the fixed mindset, people with more self-compassion can see failings or obstacles as a natural part of the learning process, not as proof that they are doomed to forever fail. In fact, when we arm our students with tools for self-compassion, we are making it more likely that they will explore more bravely and persist in the face of inevitable challenges.[21]

Part of self-kindness is as simple as it sounds: we disempower the constant internal abuse that most of us view as normal or helpful. Beyond that, it calls us to understand the hurt and harm that we cause to ourselves unnecessarily. But then it gets hard, because after we stop the self-judgment, self-compassion calls us to actively comfort ourselves, even allowing ourselves to be moved by our own pain. Neff suggests pausing to say, "This is difficult right now. How can I care for and comfort myself in this moment?"[22]

Admittedly, you cannot jump right to self-soothing with your students. For most of them, this is a mildly terrifying topic. I gave a lecture on self-compassion in my studio and needed to preface for them that the information I was providing was based on science (which somehow makes it feel safer), and I also admitted that when I first started studying self-compassion, it seemed way too hard and "out there" for me to ever make it part of my life and work.

When the voice in our heads is so critical and mean, and when *it has been our ally* in getting us as far as we've gotten, the idea of questioning it or transforming it feels so impossible as to be ridiculous. This is how insidious the problem is, and why it is so critical to share this with our students. Start small and start with the data. I still see eyes widen at the mere mention of the fact that everyone has that mean voice inside. It's freeing.

Recall that stress in our students leads to increased cortisol, which inhibits cognitive function and therefore learning. It turns out that there's a concrete way for students to address this, and it's self-kindness. When we comfort ourselves in times of stress, we trigger the release of oxytocin, the feel-good hormone that reduces fear and anxiety. Oxytocin counteracts the effects of cortisol released in times of stress. It also increases our feelings of trust, calm, and safety.[23]

Self-criticism, on the other hand, activates our old friend the amygdala, or the fear center of the brain. You'll recall this reptilian wiring from chapters 1 and 2. We detect a threat and instantly move into our programmed fight-or-flight response.[24] Studies now show that the amygdala doesn't differentiate between physical and emotional pain;[25] the physiological effects of talking to yourself harshly are the same as if you were slapped in the face. We can reduce this pain by reminding ourselves of our biological predisposition toward negativity; we can hear those thoughts and choose to focus on the good, with time and practice.

Self-Compassion in Action

There are many variations on the exercise below. I've seen a brilliant choreographer walk back and forth as though she were two characters having a disagreement. I've heard people recommend writing it out so you can see just how horrible the voice is. Neff even recommends a version where you place three chairs in a room: one for the mean voice, one for your trying self, and one for your observer self, to mediate the discussion. The essential parts are this:[26]

1. Notice when you are being self-critical. Pay attention to the actual words, tone, and so on. Get as much information as possible.
2. Try to soften the critic's voice. "I know you are trying to help but this is very hurtful."
3. Reframe the critic's commentary in the voice of your most compassionate friend.

For teachers, a great trick is to find the useful grain of sand in the commentary, and then imagine how you would reframe it for one of your students. To be successful in reframing our self-judgment, we don't need to make it go away. We begin to practice self-kindness as soon as we notice the voice berating us and realize that we have a choice.

Another useful tool recommended by Neff is a short self-compassion mantra to use whenever you are in pain. For our students, we might open the door by creating a mantra around practicing, to which they can refer when frustrations are high. To be effective, the mantra should touch on the three key components of self-compassion: giving ourselves a little bit of kindness to counteract the harsh judgment, reminding us of our common humanity (everyone feels this way), and reminding us that we have a choice about how to interact with the thought. Here are two examples from Neff, and then an adaptation I wrote. You can ask students to draft their own version and keep it on a sticky note in their binder for whenever things get hard.

> This is a moment of suffering.
> Suffering is part of life.
> May I be kind to myself in this moment.
> May I give myself the compassion I need.[27]

Another variation:

> I'm having a really hard time right now.
> Everyone feels this way sometimes. Or This is part of being human.
> May I hold my pain with tenderness. Or May I be gentle and understanding with myself.
> I am worthy of receiving self-compassion. Or I will try to be as compassionate as possible.

(Student grunts in frustration or slams piano keys)

1. Take a breath.
2. Sometimes practicing is really hard.
3. Everyone struggles with it sometimes.
4. I can learn to practice without being mean to myself.

Consent in the Voice Studio by Lauren A. Cook

> Content warning: This chapter includes discussion of fatphobia in the music and theater industries, which will involve mention of weight, size, eating disorders, dieting, and intentional weight loss. If these topics are activating for the reader, it may be wise to skip the introduction. The Best Practices section includes fewer of these aspects, but please proceed with your own self-care in mind.

Although I don't remember every detail of this moment, my body still reacts when I begin to think about it. Familiar sensations of anxiety arise—my chest tightens, my arms tingle, and I want to think about anything else.

In my junior year of college, my voice teacher was on sabbatical, and I was temporarily assigned to another teacher. He was an institution in the department, already in his seventies but with the vitality and energy of a new teacher.

It was my first experience with a male teacher, and I was already on edge, having just transferred with the intent to study with one teacher who announced her sabbatical after I had already accepted the financial aid offer. Whatever the technical reasoning was is now foggy, but my teacher asked me to step in front of the mirror. I begrudgingly acquiesced, and upon shifting position, my teacher, who must have sensed my unwillingness, remarked, "See, it's not so bad, isn't it?" A fairly innocuous comment, maybe even meant to be a compliment, but my brain and nervous system went into overdrive and panic set in. My teacher had noticed my body, perceived it, passed judgment on it. His fleeting comment was enough for my brain to spiral into the depths of wondering if he thought my body was "good" or "bad," or if he had noticed my ever-fluctuating weight, or if he thought I was attractive or not, and why did I have to be in this room on this day in this outfit with this person. Needless to say, the rest of the lesson was a blur. Always a good student, I continued to follow instructions and sing on autopilot while my brain conspired to pull me down into the depths of analyzing everything that was wrong with my body. This one comment informed me that this was no longer a neutral space, and I attended lessons for the remainder of the semester feeling tense, suspicious, afraid, and full of dread.

Part 1: What Is a Safe Space? Best Practices for Inclusivity and Consent

When I think back now on the memory above, a few questions come to mind. What would have happened if I had said no to looking in the mirror? What if this was a space where I could say "I am really struggling with my body image today and looking in the mirror fills me with dread. Is there another way to understand this concept?" What if it had already been established that sometimes looking in the mirror was activating for me, and my teacher had asked if that was something I was feeling open to doing on that day? What if I had even known that saying no to my voice teacher was an option? This small, most likely well-intentioned comment now, ten years later, brings up two major concepts that have become foundations of my teaching. First is the notion of consent in the voice studio, and how to properly create a consent-based space where teachers can encourage their students to take risks, but students also have the right to decline participation in certain pedagogical practices if they recognize it might lead to technical regression or keen activation of the nervous system. Second is identifying the elements that contribute to creating voice studios that are truly *inclusive* spaces. The fact of the matter is that these two elements are intrinsically linked, and student agency is instrumental in cultivating voice studios that are diverse and equitable.

The foundations of consent can seem both simple and complex at the same time, so it's first necessary to define the concept of a "safe" or inclusive space and what ingredients are crucial in creating one. Ultimately, for me, an inclusive space is one that considers the needs of everyone who enters it, whether they can or cannot be seen or heard. This is relevant to all facets of diversity and equity, including race, ethnicity, gender identity, disability, and body size, the last of which is often left out in inclusion efforts but is of profound importance in the performing arts. Using specific and informed language is one of the primary methods in creating these spaces, and therefore is the first ingredient.

I've chosen to name Best Practice One "Deloaded Language," a term borrowed from the work of theatrical intimacy educators Chelsea Pace and Laura Rikard. In her book *Staging Sex*, Pace describes this practice as being aware of the social and cultural contexts of certain terminology and using words that are neutral, specific, and at times, clinical.[28] In the voice studio, this would translate to using specific, anatomical terminology when referencing parts of the body. It would include honoring students' pronouns and chosen names and asking questions about their preferences regarding terminology in instances where they are not immediately clear. We only know by asking, and becoming comfortable with these questions is an important aspect of this best practice. It's imperative to note that all the best practices, including deloaded language, should be used for every student in every lesson or class. Teachers cannot predict which students may be activated by casual terminology, nor should they assume that only certain groups have this sensitivity. Likewise, teachers cannot predict which specific words may trigger a stress response but using deloaded language consistently and mindfully is a likely way to minimize negative reactions. The benefits increase when students feel empowered to voice any possible concerns regarding language and terminology, which can be a result of the next topic, Best Practice Two: Consent Based Communication.

The pillars of consent, particularly in academic environments or in situations with an uneven power dynamic (here, that of teacher and student), are quite a bit more nuanced than a simple "yes," or "no." My favorite comprehensive definition of consent uses the acronym FRIES: Freely given, Reversible, Informed, Enthusiastic, and Specific.[29] Each of these has relevance in the voice studio, and I'll briefly explain each one with scenarios most teachers will encounter at some point in their careers. First is "freely given," or uncoerced. This pillar is especially important in academic voice programs where students are being graded. Feeling as though they cannot say no to requests or suggestions for fear of grade reduction creates a coercive environment. A great way to ensure consent is freely given is to create a syllabus or studio policies that have clear and consistent grading methods and asking students to verify in writing they have read and understood them.

The remaining pillars likewise have many applications but can be clearly illustrated in regard to instructional touch, a technique many voice teachers use particularly when adjusting alignment, breath, or dealing with physical inefficiencies. For example, a simple hands-on neck adjustment might improve alignment and relieve tension in the accessory muscles of the neck.[30] This is a rather simplistic instance, but helpful, nonetheless. The "reversible" pillar would mean that even though a student has consented to this adjustment in one lesson, they can change their mind in following lessons or even later in the same one. (Note here that a student never needs to provide a reason for this. They may do so voluntarily, but if they do not, we must assume their boundary is in place for a reason.)[31] "Informed" means the student knows exactly what the instructional touch will involve—is it a slow pull back of the neck? Is the student allowing you to move the neck freely? Being careful to include these details before asking for consent ensures the response is informed. Next, "enthusiastic" consent refers to all of those additional and perhaps nonverbal signs voice teachers become so adept at reading. If the student says yes but their body language says no, the consent is not enthusiastic. While a student might not jump up and down with excitement in response to this prospect of instructional touch, the nuances of communication are important here and worth noting in these instances. If, for example, the student says yes but you can see any part of their body stiffen, or their face goes slack, or they get a faraway look in their eyes, the real answer is no. The last pillar, "specific," is what I consider the *why* of instructional touch. "Informed" provides the how and "specific" provides the reasoning. A simple statement of your pedagogical purpose here is all it takes. When used together, these pillars have the added benefit of challenging our creativity and intention. If we are encouraging students to ask "why," then we better have a good reason for the use of touch. In the long run, this reduces auto-pilot teaching and encourages deep thinking.

There are several questions I receive when discussing consent with teachers in the performing arts, and the most common is how to know if students are taking advantage of the consent-based communication by claiming they don't feel "safe" or revoking consent simply for the sake of not wanting to do a certain exercise. I try to challenge these concerns in a few ways. First, when dealing with Best Practice One, Deloaded Language, one of the principles is to use such language for all students in every lesson without assuming who might be more sensitive to certain terminology. This is also true for consent-based communication. We cannot assume who does or does not mind being touched, nor do we know what exercises are going to create a negative reaction. I don't think anyone would have guessed "simply" looking in the mirror was emotionally triggering for me. Therefore, it is entirely possible that one student out of many may set a boundary with an ulterior motive of wanting to avoid work or a new concept. For every one of those, however, there are many more students who will benefit from these practices, and I believe that minimizing negative experiences for most students that could impede future progress is worth the one or two who may misuse the principles. Keep in mind that if a student has a personal history of their boundaries being violated by another (especially by a person in authority), they may be the *least* likely to voice their concern, unless you have already taken steps to establish safety in less-activating circumstances.

Secondly, this addresses the topic of comfort versus safety. There are many occasions when the material artists work with is not comfortable. Students may need to be in roles where their characters are villains or victims of traumatic experiences. They will say lines that are in conflict with their values or tap into emotions that have been previously deeply controlled. Therefore, asking for consent in relation to whether something is comfortable may not be the most accurate phrasing. Safety, however, is mandatory. Therefore, using questions that begin with "How would it work with your boundaries if . . . " or "How would you feel if . . . " can offer a more specific representation of the work at hand, particularly when it involves a challenge or supervised risk taking.

You'll notice that all the example phrases above are open-ended questions requiring more than a one-word answer. This is imperative in creating a culture of consent especially where there is a noticeable power imbalance in the room, as is the case for most teacher-student relationships. In these situations, most students have been conditioned to feel that there is an implied "yes" to any question a teacher, conductor, or director asks, and that saying "no" will give them a reputation of being difficult or hard to work with. In easing students into a new space where saying no is acceptable, offering the suggestion of "no, but" can be helpful. An example using instructional touch can be helpful here as well. Perhaps a teacher wants to place their hands on a student's back to feel rib expansion and asks a beautifully open-ended question using the FRIES principles. The teacher might say, "I'd like to place my hands on your back while you breathe so I can get a feel for your rib expansion. How would you feel about that?" This gives the student plenty of time to truly think about their answer instead of giving an instant affirmative response. It also provides both teacher and student with options. The student might say, "I would prefer not to do that but is there something else that is similar?" or "I'd prefer not, but I'd be happy to watch you demonstrate." In this way, the student can say no, but in a way that continues the conversation and allows them to understand the concept. Like deloaded language, these moments require teachers to think on their feet and find other methods to explain concepts instead of relying on only tried-and-true methods. The benefit is then twofold—students are respected and heard, and our pedagogical approaches constantly grow and evolve, ultimately making us better teachers.

There is one additional scenario in which consent plays a critical role in student agency, and this is in group classes, masterclasses, or studio classes, particularly those in which students are providing their peers with feedback. At one point or another, most of us have been the audience to or the target of a peer giving unsolicited advice or using feedback opportunities inappropriately. Regardless of whether there is ill intent, consent-based communication tools can and should be utilized here. Teachers in this scenario must either explicitly state the guidelines of feedback and/or be prepared to step in when they are forgotten. Some teachers prefer for peers to give only positive feedback and the teacher provides points for improvement. Others will curate appropriate topics for feedback—dramatic expression only, perhaps, and not vocal technique. Others may allow students to state what they are looking for feedback on before performing, thus eliminating any commentary that is more hurtful than helpful.[32] Taking these small steps not only ensures that these classes provide students with the assessments that are most helpful to them but also instructs less experienced artists in crucial aspects of professional interaction. Additional tools for teacher feedback are found in chapter 7.

The third and final best practice is one that requires self-reflection and often stirs up discomfort on the part of the instructor and is therefore best saved for last. Best Practice Three is Challenging Implicit Bias, which aims to broaden the teacher's own views of diversity, thereby allowing them to shape their teaching methods, studio policies, and interaction with students in a manner that best aligns with inclusivity and equity. Fortunately, there are a number of resources available to educators that address methods of identifying bias, and most agree that the first step is to cultivate awareness of the bias or biases. Asking questions is a straightforward way to do this, specifically considering your impressions of students when they walk into the studio for the first time. Any judgment stemming from a superficial visual assessment of the student could be motivated by bias. For example, before a student has spoken or sung, do you make assumptions about their voice based on physical appearance, name, or clothing? Any of those preconceived notions are worth examining. Once awareness has been cultivated, however, the next step is to research literature that challenges these beliefs. Academic journals are a good place to start, as they provide peer reviewed evidence that can provoke new ways of thinking. These can be scientific, sociological, political, or economic—anything that facilitates deep understanding and creates new curiosity surrounding our rush to judgment. Part 2 below will demonstrate the process of using these best practices to create an inclusive space that is particularly focused on the issues of body diversity, physical appearance, and how to effectively instruct students who may be struggling with these elements.

Part 2: Our Bodies, Our Voices: Body Diversity as an Element of Inclusivity—Lauren A. Cook

In 2004, Covent Garden fired American dramatic soprano Deborah Voigt for being too fat to appear in their production of *Ariadne auf Naxos*. The reasons Ms. Voigt and her agent received were varied—she couldn't fit into the predesigned costume, she couldn't do the active staging, the director changed his vision.[33] Regardless of these justifications, the event sent a strong and clear message to singers: no matter how talented you are, no matter how prepared, or collegial, companies can break their contracts if they don't like how you look.

While other instances of size discrimination in the performing arts industry may have less attention, they are insidious and widespread. In a 2021 article for *The Middle Class Artist*, journalist and singer Zach Finkelstein revealed a pattern of fatphobia and weight discrimination in comments and feedback artists received during the final rounds of the Metropolitan Opera National Competition, reaching back as far as 2009 if not earlier.[34] This behavior is not limited to classical music, nor is it reserved for artists in larger bodies. In the winter of 2020, I completed a series of interviews and surveys with singers of all genres, ability level, ages, and sizes, asking them several questions about their body image and how it has affected their careers. Sixty-two percent of singers responded that their own body image had affected their careers. Furthermore, 63 percent reported that their perceptions of others' opinions about their bodies had affected their career. Almost every artist I spoke with had a negative memory of being told something was wrong with their body—too large, too tall, not the right shape, not the right look. Regardless of the numbers, these stories alone illustrate that the performing arts industry has a serious problem with fatphobia and embracing body diversity.

There are two things of note here. First, although some singers reported feedback that their bodies were too skinny or too lanky—and these comments and their effects are just as valid—the overwhelming majority were singers who were criticized for being in bodies that were too large. The world around us is an entirely anti-fat environment, and therefore, although the following application of the best practices applies to common misconceptions regarding people in larger bodies, it is certainly true that smaller figures are also frequently stigmatized.

Secondly, because most of my interviews were related to how singers were noticing and processing their body image in voice lessons, it's clear that not all the feedback is coming from producers, directors, and industry gatekeepers. Bias is also present in the voice studio, and the process below will specifically address these issues as they arise in a pedagogical environment. Additionally, even when bias is not present, it is still imperative to teach in a body neutral manner due to the myriad ways the body can be the source of emotional trauma.

Often when we recognize the source of trauma or stress, our first instinct is to avoid the wound and hope it heals itself. Unfortunately for singers, the body is not something that can be avoided. Biomechanics of breath, posture and alignment, resonance shaping, and articulator efficiency are all topics that require identification and analysis of various anatomical structures. This is a perfect opportunity for the utilization of Best Practice One, Deloaded Language. It's clear that much of our anatomy has been victim to loaded language, or what Chelsea Pace would again describe as words that have "social and cultural context."[35] Slang and factually questionable terminology both have disadvantages, being simultaneously unspecific and potentially judgmental or activating. While seemingly innocent, the word "belly" might signal to a student that the teacher has observed they carry weight in their middle, or that "a belly" is bad and the midsection should be toned and flat. Additionally, where does the belly begin? Is it just the surface around the navel? Does it start at the solar plexus and end below the navel? In contrast, the term "front center of the abdomen" is specific, factually accurate, and a nonjudgmental term. Teachers needn't be medical-level anatomists to use deloaded language. Torso, abdomen, clavicle, sternum—all of these are perfectly acceptable and do not require an advanced degree. Using this new language in the studio can be difficult, especially for teachers who have already had long careers, and it's probable that one colloquial term here and there isn't going to traumatize students for the rest of their lives. However, using deloaded language is a simple replacement for the terminology of our fore-teachers, and it is better to make small changes than risk causing long term emotional damage.

Discussing the body and making adjustments in voice lessons is also an opportunity to use consent-based practices, and this is particularly crucial in regard to instructional touch. The main element here is to ensure that students know they can refuse instructional touch without consequences, whether in the quality of your teaching, your demeanor, or grading system. Using open-ended, specific questions with no implied answer are of utmost importance here. Think of the difference between "Can I touch your stomach real fast?" and "I'd like you to place your hand over mine on your abdomen as you inhale. How would that work for you?" Sure, one takes a little longer, but it provides the student time to give an informed answer and, if possible, suggest a "no, but . . . " option. I will be the first to admit that sometimes I think, "I've known this student forever, we have done this before, does it really matter how I ask?" The answer to my mental dialogue is always yes. It is worth it. It is worth it not only in your studio and your teaching, but so that your students expect this type of instruction and direction in all facets of their lives. The empowering effects of informed consent cannot be overstated, and as we build confident singers, we build confident humans who will demand respect from a fickle and at times treacherous industry.

We've arrived now at Best Practice Three, Challenging Implicit Bias, and it is in this area of the work that I have received the most suspicion and pushback. All I ask is that you keep an open mind as I apply this practice to challenging bias toward body size and body diversity. One of the things that teachers experience in cultivating awareness of bias is feelings of discomfort and often guilt. I encourage you, if these emotions arise, to allow yourself to feel them without judgment. Implicit bias stems from evolutionary survival concepts, or that of an "us versus them" mentality that kept earlier social groups alive. However, research reports that our biases can be overcome with mindfulness and intention.[36] In my experience, the best way to cultivate awareness is to ask the difficult questions that we perhaps have been avoiding. Here are a few examples that apply directly to the realm of body diversity:

- Do I only ask "lifestyle" questions to students in larger bodies? (Cardiovascular health, acid reflux, etc.)
- Am I exploring everything this student's voice can do, or am I assigning repertoire based on body type?
- Am I encouraging students of the same caliber to pursue the same professional opportunities, regardless of how they look?
- Have I assumed this student is unhealthy because of how they look?

This is often where teachers will state, "I am not judging my students for how they look, but I have a right to be worried about their health!" It is natural to be concerned about a student's health, not just as it relates to their singing, but their overall existence. This, however, is another belief that needs to be challenged—the belief that there is an association between visual appearance and health.

If you think back to the Best Practices section, you'll recall that the second step in challenging implicit bias is finding research that facilitates the creation of new thought patterns. This is a great time to practice working through that step together. Many of us have been conditioned to believe that physical appearance and health are deeply connected, but research from as far back as 1985 in various medical and nutritional journals demonstrates that those in larger bodies do not have a shorter life expectancy than those in smaller bodies, nor are they more likely to have illnesses typically associated with weight, such as diabetes, hypertension, or cancer.[37] In fact, the evidence demonstrates that health issues for those in larger bodies are more likely to arise from the stigma surrounding weight than weight itself. This stigma can result in individuals attempting multiple extreme diets, avoiding routine healthcare, and experiencing social isolation and stress due to discrimination.[38] Additionally, eating disorder researchers have found that behaviors and symptoms of anorexia nervosa—perhaps the most infamous restrictive disorder—are just as likely to be found in people of varying body weights, and it is a gross misconception that the illness is present only in those who have the recognizable physical signs of malnourishment or emaciation.[39] In short, we have no idea if our students are healthy or not, as we are not medical practitioners, nor can our eyes determine the answer.

Let's say now that your student has disclosed that they are not, in fact, healthy. Does this student therefore not deserve your best teaching, or letters of recommendation, or roles onstage? Although there are certain instances where a student is too ill to continue voice lessons or performing, we will often have students enter our studios with thyroid abnormalities, anemia, high cholesterol, or other health issues that have no bearing on their voice.[40] This provides another opportunity for further research into any potential bias of health and worth, and most likely you will come across the Health at Every Size (HAES)® approach in this line of inquiry. The tenants of HAES® are as follows:

- Pursuing health is neither a moral imperative nor an individual obligation
- Health status should never be used to judge, oppress, or determine the value of an individual
- Accept and respect the inherent diversity of body shapes and sizes
- Reject the idealizing or pathologizing of specific weights[41]

This can be particularly tricky for teachers in the performing arts, because even once embracing or understanding the HAES® principles, the fact remains that regardless of how we advocate for diversity, equity, and inclusion of bodies of all sizes in our voice studio, the industry is a different beast. For those teaching professionals and college majors, the goal is, of course, to prepare students for the vocal and logistical challenges of the industry. In short, we want our students to get hired, and we know the industry has deep preferences for what bodies are onstage.

Even more so than challenging implicit bias, recognizing the shortcomings of our industry can be the most difficult part in the process of creating body-diverse spaces. My approach has been to make sure all students are armed with the knowledge of the realities of the business, and they can choose to go forward with the radical idea that all bodies deserve to be onstage, or they can decide this is just not their battle to fight. I respect both decisions, as I have often vacillated between the two. It is my hope, though, that by creating inclusive spaces at the training level, our students will enter the industry expecting better treatment, more rights and increased visibility than the generation before them. There are pockets of hope that change is happening. In February of 2022, for example, Brittney Johnson made history by becoming the first Black actor to take on the role of Glinda in *Wicked* full time.[42] This progress, however, must begin in the voice studio. Students must have agency over their voices, bodies, and careers, and they must be respected as humans with weaknesses, talents, emotions, and possibly even trauma. However, by using deloaded language and consent-based practices, and by continually challenging our long-held belief systems, we stand the best chance of sending confident changemakers out into a business that so desperately needs fresh perspectives.

Notes

1. Marianna Evangelia Kapsetaki and Charlie Easmon, "Eating Disorders in Musicians: A Survey Investigating Self-Reported Eating Disorders of Musicians," *Eating and Weight Disorders—Studies on Anorexia, Bulimia, and Obesity* 24 (2019): 541–49, https://link.springer.com/article/10.1007/s40519-017-0414-9.

2. Heather L. Schwartz, Michelle Bongard, Erin D. Bogan, Alaina E. Boyle, Duncan C. Meyers, and Robert J. Jagers, "Social and Emotional Learning in Schools Nationally and in the Collaborating Districts Initiative," https://casel.org/sel-in-schools-nationally-and-in-the-cdi/?view=true.

3. Scott Edgar, Jacqueline Kelly-McHale, Jared Rawlings, and Tim Lautzenheiser, *Music Education and Social–Emotional Learning: The Heart of Teaching Music* (Chicago: Gia Publications, Incorporated, 2017).

4. Edgar et al., *Music Education and Social Emotional Learning*, 12–13.

5. Ibid., 85–90.

6. Sauerland, William. "Sound Teaching." The Choral Journal 62, no. 3 (2021): 32–44.

7. Diane Poole Heller, *The Power of Attachment: How to Create Deep and Lasting Intimate Relationships* (Boulder, CO: Sounds True, 2019), 70–71.

8. Poole Heller, *The Power of Attachment*, 72–73.

9. Marc Brackett, "The Colors of Our Emotions," Marc Brackett, Ph.D., January 19, 2020, https://www.marcbrackett.com/the-colors-of-our-emotions/.

10. Poole Heller, *The Power of Attachment*, 85.

11. Cara P. Lemieux, "Brené Brown Talks to the Shriver Report: The Power of Shame on Women Living on the Brink," The Shriver Report, February 5, 2014, https://shriverreport.org/how-to-overcome-shame-when-on-the-brink-brene-brown/.

12. Kristin Neff, *Self-Compassion: The Proven Power of Being Kind to Yourself* (New York: William Morrow, 2011), 90.

13. Ibid., 19.

14. Ibid., 24.

15. Ibid., 26, 33.

16. Ibid., 110.

17. Ibid., 116.
18. Ibid., 112.
19. Ibid., 124.
20. Ibid., 123.
21. Ibid., 170.
22. Ibid., 42.
23. Ibid., 49.
24. Ibid., 82.
25. Naomi Eisenberger, Matthew Lieberman, and Kipling Williams, "Does Rejection Hurt? An fMRI Study of Social Exclusion," *Science* (New York, 2003), 302, 290–92, doi:10.1126/science.1089134.
26. Neff, *Self-Compassion*, 52–53.
27. Ibid., 119.
28. Chelsea Pace, *Staging Sex* (New York: Routledge, 2014), 11.
29. "Sexual Consent," Planned Parenthood, https://www.plannedparenthood.org/learn/relationships/sexual-consent. Accessed March 11, 2021.
30. In these instances, teachers should be using open-ended questions before offering adjustments. More on open-ended questions and power dynamics can be found in chapters 7 and 10.
31. Pace, *Staging Sex*, 15.
32. For an excellent resource on curating feedback sessions that also provides sample dialogue, see Liz Lerman and John Borstel's *Liz Lerman's Critical Response Process* (Tacoma Park, MD: Liz Lerman Dance Exchange, 2003).
33. Deborah Voigt, *Call Me Debbie* (New York: HarperCollins, 2015), 210.
34. Zach Finkelstein, "Fat-Shaming. Bullying. Is Anyone Protecting Our Young Singers?" *The Middle Class Artist*, April 5, 2021, https://www.middleclassartist.com/post/fat-shaming-bullying-is-anyone-protecting-our-young-singers.
35. Pace, *Staging Sex*, 10.
36. Daniel A. Yudkin and Jay Van Bavel, "The Roots of Implicit Bias," Opinion, *The New York Times*, December 9, 2016, https://www.nytimes.com/2016/12/09/opinion/sunday/the-roots-of-implicit-bias.html.
37. Bacon, Linda, and Lindo Bacon. Health at every size: The surprising truth about your weight. BenBella Books, Inc., 2010.
38. Ibid., 130–31.
39. K. Eiring, T. Wiig Hage, and D. L. Reas, "Exploring the Experience of Being Viewed as 'Not Sick Enough': A Qualitative Study of Women Recovered from Anorexia Nervosa or Atypical Anorexia Nervosa," *Journal of Eating Disorders* 9, no. 142 (2021): https://doi.org/10.1186/s40337-021-00495-5.
40. This of course does not apply to vocal pathology. If your student has a diagnosed vocal pathology, please follow the treatment plan in place as devised by an otolaryngologist, speech-language pathologist, or singing voice specialist.
41. "The Health at Every Size® (HAES®) Approach," Association for Size Diversity and Health, https://sizediversityandhealth.org/health-at-every-size-haes-approach/. Accessed: March 19, 2021.
42. Andrew Gans, "Watch Brittney Johnson Make History in Broadway's *Wicked*," Broadway News, *Playbill*, February 15, 2022, https://playbill.com/article/watch-brittney-johnson-make-history-in-broadways-wicked.

10

An Exploration of Vocal Dignity

Megan Durham and Emma Lynn Abrams

Certainly there are very real differences between us. But it is not those differences between us that are separating us. It is rather our refusal to recognize those differences.

—Audre Lorde

WHEN SPEAKING OF SINGING, especially teaching and learning to sing, each of us enters the conversation carrying particular histories. We also bring contexts of learning that shape our relationship to the practice and performance of singing, the contemporary music industry, and genres that we study. We would like to acknowledge the structural and behavioral ways that *dignity* is withheld from singers, identify the harm this causes, and offer constructive ideas for creating new rhythms that contribute to a musical ecosystem that recognizes *dignity* as a fundamental human right. This is an interactive chapter, so we encourage you to grab a writing utensil and spend a few moments with these preparatory reflection questions:

> How have my unique differences—as a human and a singer—been seen, validated, and respected (or not) in musical spaces?
>
> Have there been times where I have sacrificed my dignity for safety and/or survival in musical contexts?
>
> How does my lived experience of and access to *dignity* correlate to my access to power and privilege?
>
> How does my body respond to saying the word *no*? How does my body respond to receiving the word *no*?

How does my body respond to saying the word *yes*? How does my body respond to receiving the word *yes*?

The word *dignity* was rarely heard in the environments that shaped our own music education. However, it frequently emerges in the scholarship of somatic educators, civil rights advocates, and intellectuals such as Bobbie Harro, bell hooks, Audre Lorde, Sonya Renee Taylor, Kai Cheng Thom, adrienne maree brown, and Betty Martin. We are grateful to these leaders as we offer a framework for trauma-informed and anti-oppressive voice teaching, and we hope it will be supportive and clarifying for you and your students.

We acknowledge that the ideas and questions generated in these pages extend beyond the scope of one chapter and humbly offer them as a launching pad for inquiry, curiosity, and change. We also acknowledge that we are white, cisgender women, embodying multiple privileges like access, wellness, class, homeownership, education, and ability. It is our intention to continue learning, decolonizing, and community building, even as we will never be fully conscious of how often we have taken *dignity* for granted because of our privilege.

Dignity is a fundamental human right. We want every human being—every singing body—to be fully witnessed in both the wholeness of their mere existence and the complexity of their inevitable imperfection. When left untended, however, the experience of joyful singing can be shadowed by the impact of physical and emotional trauma, rendering us unable to engage fully in the learning and music-making process. By creating a framework for understanding these vulnerabilities, voice educators can develop needed support structures, provide accommodation, and co-create the culture of care needed to help each singing body thrive on their chosen path.

As teachers of singing, it is likely that we fundamentally align on this point: each singing voice is *inherently* worthy of reverence. However, many singers self-report numerous occasions in both higher education and the music industry where they felt their dignity diminished by oppressive structures, overt and covert biases, actions taken by those in positions of power, or a lack of access to compassionate support. We seek your allyship in service to actively building a culture of care in voice communities that allows dignity to thrive.

A note before we begin: we offer a number of invitations to participate in somatic practice throughout this chapter. We encourage each reader to lean into any discomfort that arises from these practices with presence and curiosity. Worship of the written word is an aspect of white body supremacy culture.[1] Even within this chapter, it is our intention to disrupt the norms of disembodied whiteness by acknowledging our bodies and the space they take up as we engage with this material.

Opening Practice

Let's begin by noticing.
Are you sitting or standing?
What is the temperature in the room?
What colors and textures do you see or sense around you? Name a few.
What do you sense inside of you? Can you name images, textures, or sensations you are present to?
All of you is welcome.
Is there anything that would make you feel more comfortable in this moment?
What is it like to first notice and then take actionable steps toward making yourself more comfortable?

When you feel ready, begin:

Breathe into the word, *dignity*. Notice how it lands in your mind, in your body, in your awareness.
Identify your response: Do you feel yourself open, shift, settle, activate, or remain neutral?
Get specific: Are there any colors, images, or additional words that come up for you when you breathe into the word, *dignity*?
Take a moment again to jot down a few of your noticings about how this word lands in your body. Write, draw, or sketch your initial response.

Use all the time you need or desire with this practice. When you are ready, bring your awareness back to this text and continue reading.

What Is "Dignity?"

The Oxford definition of *dignity* is *the state or quality of being worthy of honor or respect; a composed or serious manner or style; a sense of pride in oneself; self-respect*. This exploration seeks to contextualize dignity not only as it is defined intellectually, but also as it may be assimilated somatically. Perhaps *dignity*, like *safety*, is something that we can only truly understand through embodied experience. For example, we don't "think" safety, we "feel" it.

> *My own lived experience of singing in this body, with this voice, has led me to believe that dignity can be slippery—hard to grasp, difficult to experience, difficult to maintain, and complex in relationship to the people I love and respect, the spaces that I operate within, and the lived experience and histories I carry in my body. I can offer myself dignity through practice and clarity of intention, but I cannot guarantee it.* —Emma

It is critical to consider dignity not only individually, but also transpersonally. We all yearn for and are biologically wired to seek companionship, validation, and belonging. We can cultivate a presence that offers dignity to those around us, sending the grounded message *I am worthy of taking up space, I do not have to achieve to deserve, AND your dignity is not diminished by mine.*

Thus, we might come to understand dignity as an embodied knowing that worth is not related to binary structures. My capacity, ability, resilience, weakness, gifts, contributions, shortcomings, and the particular ways that I move, speak, sing, think, react, and inhabit space are vital because I breathe, not because I earn. My value depends on no one's estimation, and yet, my worth is intimately tied to celebrating yours.[2] Dignity depends on our mutual, collective freedom—the reclamation of one voice is bound to the liberation of all voices.

Based on your observations in the opening practice, how might you define *dignity*?

Voicework Practice (2–5 mins.)

Begin humming with lips loosely touching on any comfortable pitch in your mid-range. When you feel ready, bring to mind the word *dignity*, and allow yourself to express whatever tone qualities arise, without judgment. All sounds are welcome, including wilder or weaker sounds you may have historically been denied access to in the context of western classical voice study. If you feel pain, pause, and shift your approach.

After a while of free sound-making, close your lips and return to humming, and close the practice by presencing gratitude: for this voice, this body, for this opportunity for vocal expression.

When Dignity Is Denied

> *I want there to be a place in the world where people can engage in one another's differences in a way that is redemptive, full of hope and possibility. Not this "In order to love you, I must make you something else" That's what domination is all about, that in order to be close to you, I must possess you, remake and recast you.*
>
> —bell hooks, "Reel to Real: Race, Sex, and Class at the Movies"[3]

Dignity honors difference. If we understand this foundational axiom, we must also recognize how bias, social conditioning, and other forms of oppression impede its ability to flourish as a universal human right. It is inherent; and yet, while we may unconsciously offer it to bodies (and voices) that the societal majority idealizes, it takes conscious effort to break socialized patterns of dominance in order to offer dignity to bodies, to voices, that do not fall under normalized standards of "worth." Bobbie Harro offers insight into this phenomenon in her Cycle of Socialization theory. The author writes,

> [W]e are each born into a specific set of social identities [which] predispose us to unequal roles in the dynamic system of oppression. We are then socialized by powerful sources in our worlds to play the roles prescribed by an inequitable social system. This socialization is pervasive (coming from all sides and sources), self-perpetuating (intradependent), and often invisible (unconscious and unnamed).... We are born into a world with the mechanics of oppression already in place. We have no consciousness, no choice, no blame, no guilt. There is no information or, limited information, or misinformation about social identity and power. Bias, stereotyping, prejudice, habits, tradition, and a history of oppression already exist. We inherit them without our permission.[4]

The cycles that Harro identifies prevent dignity from thriving, especially in bodies that have been marginalized within a system that is designed for the comfort of white, cis, and able bodies with material and social access and unconditional respect. As we consider this within the voice context, we might ask, how have voice systems (i.e., university programs, young artist programs, opera houses, voice studios, K–12 music education, etc.) entrained participants into an often unconscious cycle of repression?

Our collective answers to this question would likely reflect innumerable ways that Western classical voice culture has perpetuated systemic oppression—and it is beyond the scope of this chapter to unmask them all. Instead, in an attempt to right the wrongs of previous generations, we might center the question: *Who has power?*

Much has been written about the various types of power, particularly the differences between *power-over* (dominance, control, and manipulation) and *power-with* (collaboration, co-creation, and mutual respect). In her book *Truth or Dare*, author and activist Starhawk writes,

> *Power-over* is the power of the prison guard, of the gun, power that is ultimately backed by force[;] ... *power-with* is the power of a strong individual in a group of equals, the power not to command, but to suggest and be listened to, to begin something and see it happen[;] ... *power-from-within* arises from our sense of connection, our bonding with other human beings, and with the environment.[5]

Historically, voice pedagogy has operated in *power-over* paradigms.[6] In this model, the master teacher assumes full control and knowledge of a student's singing body, often dictating the student's experience to them rather than asking the student to describe their own experience (i.e., "You should feel XYZ happen when you do X"). In this dominance-based approach, singers can shut down, dissociate, and internalize shame when exercises are not "properly" executed. It is implicitly understood that the purpose of walking into a voice lesson is to *get better*, to be *corrected*, to be somehow different than we currently are—that voice work operates in the context of assumed deficiency. Even the word "lesson" has dual meanings: *to instruct or teach, and/or to admonish and rebuke*. The long-term impacts of learned helplessness due to a lack of pedagogical clarity, constant shaming, and chronic disempowerment can be psychologically devastating. Over time, singers can perceive themselves to feel *owned by* and *obligated to* a particular method, person, or institution, rather than trusting their own experiences, embodied responses, and choices as sovereign beings.

When participating in educational relationships that cultivate a *power-with* dynamic, singers instead learn that they can be active participants in an emergent, co-creative learning process. Teachers embodying this approach help singers to recognize that what they are looking for already exists within them and offer choice-based strategies toward acquiring needed skills. Dignity flourishes when we engage in p*ower-with* pedagogy that ultimately cultivates *power-from-within*—the ability to connect with our innate goodness and reciprocally participate in communities of care. In short, we shift toward a sustainable model of *assumed wholeness*.

It is likely that many of the singing environments that you have participated in have demonstrated *power-over* dynamics. Much of this can be attributed to the historical roots of the Western Classical tradition—an art form birthed within the context of seventeenth and eighteenth century aristocracies; Western Classical Music has foundations in appeasing the tastes of ruling classes. This structure persists into the modern era in the context of late capitalism through relational dynamics with wealthy donors, pay-to-sing performance opportunities, board politics within arts organizations, and conscious and unconscious gatekeeping.

One specific way that the *power-over* (or "master") paradigm often manifests is through the emergence of voice teacher as "hero" or "rescuer" persona. When a voice teacher positions themselves as the hero/enabler, students may find themselves disempowered and have difficulty accessing agency. This form of paternalism perpetuates the idea that without a teacher's guidance (power), the student (stripped of autonomy) will be unable to perform at a particular level. In this model, the teacher becomes the sole authority for vocal health, beauty, freedom, and so forth, disempowering students to define their own experiences or take appropriate credit for successes or failures.

Many of us have internalized messages around this common archetype in singing spaces. The "rescuer identity" in voice contexts may sound like:

> If I have the right training, I will be able to "fix" my students.
> Knowledge of my body equates to knowledge of all bodies.
> Without my guidance, my students would feel lost.
> No other teacher can reach this student like me.
> I am solely responsible for the performance outcomes of my students.
> My self-worth is tied to my ability to teach.
> I cannot bear the idea of someone leaving my studio.
> The students I work with are fragile.

Offering ourselves compassion, can we notice this archetype if it emerges? Can we learn to sit with discomfort when we don't have an answer, resisting the urgency to "fix?" Resting in the truth that our knowledge is valuable, and yet we are not the authority of our students' singing bodies, can we affirm and embody that our self-worth does not depend on our ability to "save" singing voices?

Affirmations for rescuer tendencies may sound like:

- Voices are not fragile. Voices are resilient.
- All singing bodies are capable, creative, and able to make their own choices.
- I can help students become their own teacher.
- My self-worth does not depend on my ability to teach.
- I honor both my knowledge and the students' lived experiences.
- I am only in charge of my singing body.
- My role is to offer choices, not impose fixes.
- My voice is not a project; students are not projects; my body is not a project.

Power-over dynamics in voice culture might also manifest through body policing. Performance industries epitomize the "ideal" singing body, as if fitness or aesthetic goals should mirror singing goals. This maintains the false and capitalistic narrative that body shape, health, wellness, and size is a choice we can all make through hard work, discipline, and self-control. In this paradigm, it is *your fault* if your "bad or undisciplined choices" impact your voice through things like weight gain, acid reflux, or vocal fatigue.

Words associating voice work with athleticism like "fitness and health"[7] are often used interchangeably, undefined, and decontextualized. This can perpetuate an ableist message that equates vocal wellness with an idealized form of ability that may not be accessible or relevant for all bodies. Language can have a significant impact on how dignity is affirmed or denied in voice pedagogy. It can be particularly challenging when a word or phrase that feels beneficial for *us* as the teacher is not helpful for the *student*. The word "athlete" is one example.

Take a moment and breathe into the word: *athlete*. Notice what comes up for you. What feelings of comfort, discomfort, connection, or tightness emerge in your body? What is your body intelligence telling you? This can be a tricky word—one that may require significant reflection before applying generally, or with assumption, in voice settings. As we acknowledge its use as a potentially effective metaphor in singing contexts, can we also hold space for how it may not resonate with everyone that we work with? For some, this word signals feelings of growth, empowerment, and skill. For others, it signals shame, elitism, and disconnection.

"Athlete" can connote physical and emotional exceptionalism that may not be available. Depending on your experience with this word, it can reflect a grind-culture mentality where worth is measured by hard work, constant achievement, perfectionism, and the urgency to act, win, and compete. It may also perpetuate the colonizer belief that "healthy" or "able" bodies (voices) have greater value than other bodies (voices), which aligns with violent ideologies such as white body supremacy. It can also generate feelings of competition, scarcity, and never-enoughness. Consider the Greek etymology: "to compete for a prize" in relation to voice care. A constant emphasis on competition (in both personal and professional voice work) commodifies well-intended pedagogic principles into marketing strategies. It's easy to be sold on the idea that your voice isn't ____ enough. Body optimization sells.

This is not to suggest that we stop using this word (especially if it's meaningful for you), or refuse to honor how strength, resilience, and skill-building may be significant parts of one's process. Can we instead hold a *both/and* perspective with popular messages in voice care and performance preparation? Can we take time to intentionally reflect on how our words may be received, especially when cultivating *power-with* relationships in the voice studio?

Reflections on Power

How do you identify when you are in a power-over or power-with relationship? One way is through noticing your body's responses through somatic practice. Bring to mind a specific context in which you sing—this could be a lesson, rehearsal, or performance. Consider these questions:

> How is power held in this space and who has power? Who makes decisions?
>> Is power held by one individual or collectively shared among all musicians?
>> Does this singing space feel co-creative or corrective/coercive?
>> Imagine you receive a request from the person or people in charge.
>> Do you have access to *no* within this space? How does it feel in your body to say *no* in this space? Are there implicit or explicit consequences to saying *no*?

Do you have access to *yes* within this space? What happens if you say *yes*? Are there implicit or explicit expectations that you will say *yes*?

Voicework Practice

1. Stand up or sit comfortably.
2. Using your right arm, lightly pat or tap your left arm and become present to the sensation of your hand against your arm. You can play with the kind of touch that feels most enjoyable and comfortable to you in this moment—light pats, firm pats, fast, slow, and so on.
3. As you tune into the sensation against your skin, affirm out loud to yourself: "This is my right arm. This arm belongs to me. Thank you, arm."
4. Repeat this, changing your language for your other arm, head, throat/neck, chest, belly, back, butt, legs, and feet. Offer gratitude for each area of your body in turn.
5. When you are finished, notice if your quality of attention has shifted such that you are more present to your present moment body and skin sensations.

How can we create singing spaces that promote dignity?

Honoring Difference

Vocal dignity means honoring the intelligence of diverse bodies with individual lived experiences.

In considering the intersection of dignity and voice care, we'd like to invite you into an experiment of radical imagination: consider for a moment an expanded definition of voice that is not limited to acoustic properties or the ability to hear them.

Perhaps voice can mean any form of self-expression—from movement to primal sound making, to electronic sound making, to instrument playing, to sitting and breathing as the vibration of heartbeat and air mingle. Consider that the inner vibration of life force can be understood to be voice, or that the expression of this life force through sound or movement is a sacred act of expression.

Not every body uses vocal folds to sing; not every body uses ears to listen. There is no hierarchy of sound and silence: often the most powerful or meaningful parts of music are places of intentional silence or rest. Some voices may not always have access to sound making, whether due to illness, injury, ability, or choice, and that's okay. Vocal dignity affirms that resonance properties alone may not be a reflection of all bodies' authentic voices.

As voice teachers, it is our understanding that we learn anatomy to hold an informed space—not to simply fill space with information. Bodies are complex meetings of our physical, psychological, energetic, historical, and spiritual selves. Our task must not be simply to understand how the lungs function but to know how and to what purpose all bodies breathe. Understanding acoustic science does not give a teacher the right to presume to know how sound feels traveling through another person's physical body. Bodies are diverse lived and living experiences and our teaching must hold space for the humility of presence required to create space for this truth.

As we discussed, historical models of voice pedagogy often celebrate normative, colonial standards of beauty, style, and performance practice, which are often taught through modeling "sound hegemony"—*this vowel goes here, this breath should be here, this line should . . .* , and so forth. Even as we seek to create goals and appropriate challenges around creativity and functionality that prioritize skill building and honor the tradition from whence we come, centering vocal dignity assumes wholeness, and celebrates the diverse and unique ways that voices and bodies access sound and artistry.

As creators of voice culture, we must intentionally shift away from an "assumed deficiency" model that asks, "What needs to be corrected?" toward an "assumed wholeness" model that asks, "What needs to be nurtured?"

Celebrating Choices

We prioritize offering choices over giving answers, perhaps with the affirmation:

I am a curious and humble participant in your process. I am a guest in your physical and acoustic space.

Betty Martin, somatic sex educator and creator of the Wheel of Consent, often asks, *What are we doing, and who is it for?*[8] A critical part of cultivating choice and boundaries in a voice studio is offering permission for students to say, "No." Giving individuals the agency to create their own boundaries helps to decolonize traditional power structures where the teacher assumes total ownership and knowledge of the student's voice/body.

Practically, this might look like the following:

- No, that song does not feel comfortable for me.
- No, that technique does not resonate with me.
- No, that practice does not feel safe for me.
- No, I do not understand your instructions.

Are you offering permission for students to say *no*? Why might hearing *no* from a student feel uncomfortable? Are you attuned to your own boundaries and/or consciously aware of what *no* feels like in your own body? If we struggle with understanding what *no* feels like in our bodies, it can be difficult to offer it or to hear it from someone else. We may give off an unconscious "lack of permission"—that we are fragile and can't handle any conflict. When we are more conscious of our own *no*, we can more clearly and intentionally interact with others.

When we have experienced trauma, there is often great wisdom in not being able to say or feel into *no* because it has been a protective strategy in the past. If this has been the case for a student, offering them the chance to make choices and set boundaries helps them to know that we are sturdy leaders, that we are not fragile, and we will not leave if they say *no* to an activity. In fact, what if we celebrated *no*? When a student says *no*, they are enacting agency. It can be an interesting question to then ask, "What in your body is telling you *no*? Where do you feel that coming from?" What a beautiful, embodied gift to pause and notice *no* in the body.

This practice is inspired by the work of Jane Clapp, a somatic educator, creator of Jungian Somatics, and a Movement for Trauma educator. As with anything, please choose *not* to do this if it doesn't feel right for you at this moment.

Yes, No, Maybe Practice

Take a moment and orient toward the words *more comfortable*. What might bring more comfort? Shifting, moving, settling. If there is a place on your body that it might feel nice to touch, inviting a sense of comfort, please place your hand there. I'm going to offer a series of three words. See if or where they land in your body.

Sense into the Word "No."

Try speaking to yourself or aloud different volumes and energy levels of the word *no*: No. No, thank you. NO. NOOOOO. No. Nope. No.

Where does *no* live in your body? Is there memory attached to that word? Is there a physical sensation, color or an image coming up for you with this word?

Now Sense into the Word "Maybe."

Try speaking to yourself or aloud different volumes and energy levels of the word *maybe*: Maybe. Mayyyyybeee? Maybe.

Where does *maybe* live in your body? If it feels right, you might try speaking the word out loud.

Sense into the Word "Yes."

Try speaking to yourself or aloud different volumes and energy levels of the word *yes*: Yes. YES! Yes.

Where does *yes* land in your body? What might it feel like to say *yes* out loud?

When you are ready, bring your awareness back into your space. Notice and perhaps journal about any observations, sensations, or ideas that emerged from this practice.

Centering Both/And

We honor multiple truths about our bodies and voices.

When we have experienced chronic or traumatic stress, we may become safety-seeking at all costs. In acute threat, this strategy makes good biological sense—our body chooses the safer-seeming path. However, if we are unable to move through or process the traumatic event, we may become stuck in a hypervigilant pattern of safety seeking. People, situations, and environments are continually rated on a binary "safe or unsafe" scale, and it can become difficult to see multiple possibilities or hold multiple truths: *is this right or wrong? . . . good or bad? . . . moral or immoral? . . . shameful or pure?*

As musicians, our self-critic often lurks in these dual taunts, sitting in constant judgment of our sounds, choices, and outcomes. How might our relationships with ourselves and one another transform if we learned to be with things that are difficult from a more non-dual perspective? Can we assume the role of a witness rather than a judge of our experiences?

Non-Dual Practice

We invite you to breathe into these statements and notice how they land or move in your body. In a gesture of holding both ideas simultaneously, you might open both palms, closing the right, then left, while reading each sentence.

I am both worthy and humble.
I feel anxious when performing, and I am an empowered singer.

I can desire evidence and techniques, and also recognize that sometimes the only available tool is presence.

I experience vocal injury, and I sing from wholeness.

Singing is my lifeline, and my self-worth does not depend on my ability to perform.

Even as I learn, I already have the information that I need.

Re-sounding Joy

Resonance is an acoustic affirmation of vitality.

By honoring our differences, celebrating choices, and leaning into nonbinary narratives about our bodies and voices, we affirm that the only requirement of worthiness is breath, and that our voices are capable of pleasurable transformation. Sometimes we spend so much time focused on changing the *external* experience of our sound that we forget how the *internal* experience changes us. Vibration stimulates the vagus nerve, which invites feelings of well-being, increases our capacity and resiliency for stress, and supports our interconnectedness to self and others. Singing is an acoustic representation of aliveness, and brings us into community physically, vibrationally, and neurophysiologically. Our resonance generates joy, both psychologically and physiologically.

In the book *Pleasure Activism*, author adrienne maree brown writes,

> Pleasure is a feeling of happy satisfaction and enjoyment. Activism consists of efforts to promote, impede, or direct social, political, economic, or environmental reform or stasis with the desire to make improvements in society. Pleasure activism is the work we do to reclaim our whole, happy and satisfiable selves from the impacts, delusions, and limitations of oppression and/or supremacy.... [U]ltimately, pleasure activism is us learning to make justice and liberation the most pleasurable experiences we can have on this planet.[9]

Perhaps our ultimate desire in creating *power-with* spaces of vocal dignity is to *reclaim our whole, happy, and satisfiable selves.* How might singing with the intention to reclaim, revive, and connect become activism? Some guiding questions might include the following:

When I hear the word, "pleasure," what is the first word that comes to my mind? Color? Image? Feeling tone in my body?
　How might I define "pleasure," and is it actively part of my life?
　Are there any barriers to pleasure in my life?

How can joy support or balance experiences of anxiety, depression, and/or trauma?

What aspects of singing (and teaching singing, if applicable), do or do not provide pleasure for me?

Should "authentic singing" always feel pleasurable?

How might my singing and/or teaching of singing become a practice of justice and liberation

A Final Practice: Holding both Dignity and Humility

This practice was originally taught to me by Kai Cheng Thom.[10] *I honor her work and am grateful to pass it on.*

1. Inhale as you lift your hands above your head in any way that feels spacious.
2. Breathe in the word *dignity*.
3. Sense into this word in your body. Notice if a color or image comes to mind. Live in this space for a moment.
4. Exhale, bringing your hands down to rest on your legs, pressing into the surface.
5. Breathe into the word *humility*.
6. Sense into this word in your body. Again, noticing if an image or color comes to mind for you.
7. Inhale, coming back into your gesture of *dignity*.
8. Remember the feeling that you cultivated initially.
9. Then ask yourself: can I also find humility here? Can I bring humility into my dignity?
10. Exhale, coming back into the gesture of *humility*.
11. Remember the feeling that you cultivated initially.
12. Then ask, Can I find *dignity* here, as I am humble? Can I bring *dignity* into my *humility*?
13. On your next exhale, affirm: *I can rest in both my worth and my humility.*
14. When you are ready, bring your awareness back into your space.

I sing,
reaching into bones and matter,
remembering aliveness.
Inside and outside resonating
with the embodied recognition
that when I am heard,
I am known.

Notes

1. "Worship of the written word shows up as: an inability or refusal to acknowledge information that is shared through stories, embodied knowing, intuition and the wide range of ways that we individually and collectively learn and know; continued frustration that people and communities don't respond to written communication; blaming people and communities for their failure to respond; those with strong documentation and writing skills are more highly valued, even in organizations where ability to relate to others is key to the mission, those who write things down get recognized for ideas that are collectively and generationally informed in a context where systemic racism privileges the writing and wisdom of people in the white group; academic standards require "original" work when our knowledge and knowing almost always builds on the knowledge and knowing of others, of each other claiming "ownership" of [written] knowledge to meet ego needs rather than understanding the importance of offering what you write and know to grow and expand the community's knowing." "Worship of the Written Word," White Supremacy Culture, https://www.whitesupremacyculture.info/worship-of-written-word.html.

2. In A brief history of human dignity, author Nicole Yeatman writes,

> "Human dignity is the inherent worth of each individual human being.... But human dignity means more than the absence of violence, discrimination, and authoritarianism. It means giving individuals the freedom to pursue their own happiness and purpose—a freedom that can be hampered by restrictive social institutions or the tyranny of the majority. The liberal ideal of the good society is not just peaceful but also pluralistic: It is a society in which we respect others' right to think and live differently than we do."

"A Brief History of Human Dignity," Big Think, November 30, 2020, https://bigthink.com/the-present/what-is-human-dignity/.

3. bell hooks, *Reel to Real: Race, Class and Sex at the Movies* (New York: Routledge, 1996).

4. Maurianne Adams, *Readings in Diversity and Social Justice* (London: Routledge, 2010).

5. Starhawk, *Truth or Dare: Encounters with Power, Authority, and Mystery* (San Francisco: HarperSanFrancisco, 1988).

6. As discussed in chapter 5, in the text *Humane Music Education for the Common Good*, contributing author Emily Good-Perkins writes,

> Historically, bel canto singing was intertwined with colonialism. In nineteenth-century Britain, vocal pedagogy was referred to as "voice culture," where "culture" in the 19th century was synonymous with "civilization." The "othering" of singing voices justified the use of vocal teaching to "civilize" and refine those who were not part of white bourgeois culture for the betterment of society . . . voice culture provided the opportunity for re-forming the voice, for colonizing yet more of the other's body . . . the singing voice . . . became the vehicle for "symbolic violence."

IrisYob and Estelle R. Jorgensen (eds.), *Humane Music Education for the Common Good* (Bloomington: Indiana University Press, 2020).

7. "What most people consider 'health' is really 'fitness.' Using language like 'fit and active' to define and inform health has been a strategy to guilt and shame those of us with varying abilities around movement and mobility. While physical fitness has marked health and the likeliness of living a longer life for years, it is not the determining factor. There are so many people like my grandpa who never ran a mile a day in their life, lived to be 88, and got to die in their favorite chair. So what does healthism really do? It makes people at odds with their bodies' inability to do physical tasks, like running a mile. It makes people associate that inability with their health—or worse, their mortality. . . . And no, I'm not knocking anyone's fitness steeze. I'm saying that it's time we think a bit deeper about calling our pursuit of fitness 'healthy living.'" TaMeicka L. Clear, "Fitness and Health Are Not the Same," The Thirlby, https://www.thethirlby.com/thejournal/2019/9/15/fitness-and-health-are-not-the-same-no-matter-what-fatphobia-attempts-to-claim. Last modified September 16, 2020.

8. Betty Martin, "What Are We Doing?" BettyMartin.org, March 6, 2015, https://bettymartin.org/?sermon=introduction. Last modified, July 27, 2022.

9. See adrienne maree brown, *Pleasure Activism: The Politics of Feeling Good* (Edinburgh: AK Press, 2019).

10. Kai Cheng Thom: writer, performer, cultural worker, and speaker, http://www.kaichengthom.com.

Conclusion

Trauma Awareness as a Social Justice Practice

Emily Jaworski Koriath

Besides trauma, there is something else human beings routinely pass on from person to person and from generation to generation: resilience. Resilience is built into the very cells of our bodies. It is as much a part of us as our ability to heal.[1]

—Resmaa Menakem

WILLIAM SAUERLAND, the author of *Queering Vocal Pedagogy*, offers the following reflection:

A few years ago, a colleague of mine, Eileen, a music therapist and music therapy professor, suggested to me the idea of welcoming women in recovery from substance use disorders to join the community chorus I direct at the university. While Eileen had spent weeks providing music therapy services to these women, she noticed a desire within them to experience a more traditional form of music making. One central purpose of this collaborative initiative was to bring music therapy out of the traditional therapy space to a natural therapeutic environment in the community setting.

Including the women in the choral ensemble created an opportunity not only for them to explore group music making, but it allowed me, as the ensemble's leader, to reimagine my pedagogy. I was aware that musical vocabulary, choral traditions, and member expectations that might feel exclusionary would need to be introduced in a way that allowed new members to feel welcome in the community, while seasoned members would have a greater appreciation for their knowledge. Through a reflective practice, I aimed to improve my teaching skills to create a community where all members—no matter their musical prowess—feel seen and valued. Appreciating the distinct lived experiences of each chorister, I adopted trauma-informed pedagogy in the choral environment. Trauma-informed pedagogy is not a system to heal trauma, but a framework for care to realize, recognize, and compassionately respond to trauma and to resist re-traumatization.

The community chorus has provided a safe space for women in recovery to integrate back into the community and engage in a positive experience they may have known before addiction. Choral singing can create a community built around collaboration, togetherness, and joy. This co-vibrating and friendship-building can be soul-mending and spirit-healing. My understanding of trauma-informed care has heightened my capacity to see each chorister as a unique and special person; each of whom might be haunted by trauma. Though as a choral director I am unable to therapeutically treat their traumatic experiences, I am more adept in offering them a safer space through a trauma-informed teaching practice.

—William Sauerland

The bottom line is that our students have changed. Whether due to the agonizing pace of the world around us, or an increased awareness of conditions that require help, more singers are coming to voice work with anxiety, depression, and trauma. We as voice professionals must adapt our practices to serve these students and enable them to tap into the artistry that will shape the world for future generations. They need our partnership, not our disdain.

Minoritized individuals, in particular, need allyship in a white, heterosexual, and cisgender dominant industry. We simply must acknowledge the truth that the lived experiences of students of color, sexual minorities, and transgender students shape them as artists and humans in ways that many voice professionals will never experience. As we strive to decolonize education, the opera industry, musical theater, commercial voice, and classical music, we must honor these artists, their lives, and what they have to say about the world around us. Learning how trauma impacts all of us goes a small way toward creating the changes we wish to see. Each of us also needs to commit to examining and dismantling the biases that have been passed down to us, especially regarding which voices and bodies are perceived to have value and which are not. Pedagogy is political, and teachers of the performing arts are not immune to this fact. In an industry that is still struggling to recognize the contributions of women, there is much work to be done within each of us and in our structures at large to truly make space for the vocal dignity of all.

Trauma is not a respecter of persons, but it does disproportionately affect minoritized groups. You'll recall our brief discussion of the Adverse Childhood Experiences (ACE) study, conducted from 1995 to 1997 and including over seventeen thousand participants. Almost two thirds of those surveyed had at least one ACE. One in five respondents had three or more ACEs. Those most likely to experience multiple ACEs and higher risk for associated mental and physical health effects in adulthood included racial and ethnic minorities, sexual minorities, and individuals of lower socioeconomic status.[2] The CDC concluded that "some populations are more vulnerable to experiencing ACEs because of the social and economic conditions in which they live, work, and play."[3] These conditions, termed social determinants of health (SDOHs), disproportionately affect vulnerable populations. As defined by the U.S. Department of Health and Human Services Healthy People 2030, SDOHs are "conditions in the environments where people are born, live, learn, work, play, worship and age that affect a wide range of health, functioning and quality of life outcomes and risks."[4] The World Health Organization (WHO) has also published information about social determinants of health and asserts that these conditions are "shaped by the distribution of money, power, and resources at global, national, and local levels."[5] The WHO also states that these social determinants are the major cause of health inequities in the United States and around the world.[6]

The CDC has recently published literature summarizing a growing body of research on the profound impact of racism on health outcomes in communities of color. They note that "racial and ethnic minority groups, throughout the United States, experience higher rates of illness and death across a wide range of health conditions, including diabetes, hypertension, obesity, asthma, and heart disease, when compared to their White counterparts."[7] Racism and other forms of discrimination are SDOHs.[8] Racism is also recognized as a public health issue.[9]

One example of the disparity in health outcomes for communities of color is reported by Raj Patel and Rupa Marya in *Inflamed: Deep Medicine and the Anatomy of Injustice*, a comprehensive analysis of the countless ways that people in historically marginalized groups are primed for negative health outcomes. Patel and Marya write,

> Stress ages the brain in ways that lead to cognitive decline. The impact is dose dependent: the more stressful events you experience, the greater your degree of mental impairment will be. Which is why it's important to remember that lifetimes of stress add up differently for different communities. A stressful event can cause changes in the brain that create a permanent cognitive impairment by literally changing the architecture of neurons and the density of connectivity. . . . Black people report up to 84 percent more mean lifetime stressful events than white folks. Cumulative lifetime stress accelerates the aging of the brain.[10]

As Megan and Emma asked in chapter 10, as a vocal practitioner, how can we release the colonial roots of vocal instruction to help singers find the power *within*? How can we invite singers to be our collaborators and co-conspirators in discovery and exploration? Given what we know about racial violence in American history, it is of deep significance if a young Black student feels the authority, autonomy, and *safety* necessary to say *no* to me, a white lady in a position of perceived authority. Such an act could have resulted in death only a century ago. We will make mistakes along the way, and occasionally hurt others as we learn and grow, but we will be choosing the clean pain of striving to be better over the dirty pain of continuing to sweep harmful practices under the rugs of academia and classical music.

Notes

1. Resmaa Menakem, *My Grandmother's Hands: Racialized Trauma and the Pathway to Mending Our Hearts and Bodies* (Las Vegas: Central Recovery Press, 2017), 50.

2. Centers for Disease Control and Prevention (CDC), "About the CDC-Kaiser ACE Study," https://www.cdc.gov/violenceprevention/aces/about.html.

3. Ibid.

4. Healthy People 2030, "Social Determinants of Health," U.S. Department of Health and Human Services, https://health.gov/healthypeople/priority-areas/social-determinants-health.

5. World Health Organization (WHO), "Social Determinants of Health," https://www.who.int/westernpacific/activities/taking-action-on-the-social-determinants-of-health.

6. Ibid.

7. Centers for Disease Control and Prevention (CDC), "Racism and Health," https://www.cdc.gov/healthequity/racism-disparities/index.html.

8. Healthy People 2030, "Social Determinants of Health."

9. CDC, "Racism and Health."

10. Marya Rupa and Raj Patel, *Inflamed: Deep Medicine and the Anatomy of Injustice*, first edition (New York: Farrar Straus and Giroux, 2021), 309.

Bibliography

Andre, Naomi. *Black Opera: History, Power, Engagement.* Urbana: University of Illinois Press, 2018.

Andre, Naomi Adele, Karen M. Bryan, and Eric Saylor, eds. *Blackness in Opera.* Urbana: University of Illinois Press, 2012.

Austin, Diane. *The Theory and Practice of Vocal Psychotherapy: Songs of the Self.* London, England, United Kingdom: Jessica Kingsley Publishers, 2009.

Brackett, Marc A. *Permission to Feel: Unlocking the Power of Emotions to Help Our Kids Ourselves and Our Society Thrive.* 1st ed. New York: Celadon Books, 2019.

Brown, Brené. *Dare to Lead: Brave Work Tough Conversations Whole Hearts.* New York: Random House 2018

Caputo Rosen, Debra, Jonathan Brandon Sataloff, and Robert Thayer Sataloff. *Psychology of Voice Disorders.* 2nd ed. San Diego: Plural Publishing, 2021.

Dana, Deb. *Anchored: How to Befriend Your Nervous System Using Polyvagal Theory.* Boulder, CO: Sounds True, 2021.

Dweck, Carol. *Mindset: The New Psychology of Success* New York: Ballantine Books, 2007.

Eustis, Lynn. *The Singer's Ego: Finding Balance Between Music and Life: A Guide for Singers and Those Who Teach and Work with Singers.* Chicago,: GIA Publications, Inc., 2005.

Eustis, Lynn. *The Teacher's Ego: When Singers Become Voice Teachers* Chicago: GIA Publications, Inc., 2013.

Gottlieb, Lori. *Maybe You Should Talk to Someone: A Therapist, Her Therapist, and Our Lives Revealed.* Boston: Houghton Mifflin Harcourt, 2019.

Haines, Staci. *The Politics of Trauma.* Berkeley: North Atlantic Books. 2019.

Helding, Lynn. *The Musician's Mind: Teaching, Learning, and Performance in the Age of Brain Science.* Lanham, MD: Rowman & Littlefield Publishers, 2020.

Levine, Peter A., and Ann Frederick. *Waking the Tiger: Healing Trauma: The Innate Capacity to Transform Overwhelming Experiences*. Berkeley: North Atlantic Books, 1997.
Lipsky, Laura van Dernoot, Connie Burk, and Jon R Conte. *Trauma Stewardship: An Everyday Guide to Caring for Self While Caring for Others*. 1st ed. Oakland, CA: Berrett-Koehler, 2009.
Marya, Rupa, and Raj Patel. *Inflamed: Deep Medicine and the Anatomy of Injustice*. 1st ed. New York: Farrar Straus and Giroux, 2021.
Menakem, Resmaa. *My Grandmother's Hands: Racialized Trauma and the Pathway to Mending Our Hearts and Bodies*. Las Vegas: Central Recovery Press, 2017.
Neff, Kristin. *Self-Compassion: The Proven Power of Being Kind to Yourself*. New York: William Morrow, 2011.
Poole Heller, Diane. *The Power of Attachment: How to Create Deep and Lasting Intimate Relationships*. Boulder, CO: Sounds True, 2019.
Rawlings, Jared, Jacqueline Kelly-McHale, and Scott Edgar. *Music Education and Social Emotional Learning: The Heart of Teaching Music*. Chicago: Gia Publications, Incorporated, 2017.
Ristad, Eloise. *A Soprano on Her Head: Right-Side-Up Reflections on Life and Other Performances*. Lafayette, CA: Real People Press, 1981.
Sauerland, William. *Queering Vocal Pedagogy: A Handbook for Teaching Trans and Genderqueer Singers and Fostering Gender-Affirming Spaces*. Lanham, MD: Rowman & Littlefield Publishers, 2022.
Savvidou, Paola. *Teaching the Whole Musician: A Guide to Wellness in the Applied Studio*. New York: Oxford University Press, 2021.
Taylor, Sonya Renee. *The Body Is Not an Apology: The Power of Radical Self-Love*. Oakland, CA: Berrett-Koehler, 2018.
Van der Kolk, Bessel A. *The Body Keeps the Score: Brain Mind and Body in the Healing of Trauma*. New York: Penguin Books, 2015.
Yob, Iris, and Estelle R. Jorgensen, eds. *Humane Music Education for the Common Good*. Bloomington: Indiana University Press, 2020.

Index

ableism, 76, 80, 191
abuse, 76, 81, 90, 94, 105, 110, 126, 137
ACDA (American Choral Directors' Association), 163–64
ACEs (Adverse Childhood Experiences), xxii, 3–4, 52, 90, 202–3
The Actor's Secret (Polatin), ix
addiction, 58, 126, 144, 148, 202
adrenaline, xvi, 9, 12, 19, 34, 77, 144
Adult Attachment Interview Protocol (George, Kaplan and Main), 52
Adverse Childhood Experiences (ACEs), xxii, 3–4, 52, 90, 202–3
Affective Development in Infancy (Brazelton and Yogman), 57
affirmations, for rescuers, 191
agency, 76, 79, 82, 83, 167, 190, 194; challenge and, 115; student, 152, 174, 178, 183, 195
The Age of Overwhelm (van Dernoot Lipsky), 147
Ainsworth, Mary, xxi, 49–50, 57
Alexander, Frederick Matthias, ix
Alexander Technique, ix, xiv, 123, 168
ambivalent (anxious) attachment, 50, 56–57, 59, 70, 157, 166–67

American Choral Directors' Association (ACDA), 163–64
American Psychiatric Association, xiii
American Psychological Association (APA), 100, 105, 110, 114
American Speech-Language-Hearing Association (ASHA), 30, 96–98, 100, 103–4, 112–13
amygdala, 18–20, 94, 131, 145, 172
Anchored (Dana), 43, 109, 146
André, Naomi, 136
ANS. *See* autonomic nervous system
anxious (ambivalent) attachment, 50, 56–57, 59, 70, 157, 166–67
APA (American Psychological Association), 100, 105, 110, 114
aphonia, 34, 39, 65
artistry, xiv–xv, 78, 84
The Artist's Way (Cameron), 107
The Artist's Way at Work (Cameron), 108
ASHA (American Speech-Language-Hearing Association), 30, 96–98, 100, 103–4, 112–13
"athlete," 192, 200n7

attachment adaptation: anxious, 50, 56–57, 59, 70, 157, 166–67; avoidant, 50, 53–56, 59, 156–57, 164–65; awareness of, 57–58; disorganized, 50, 57–60, 167; insecure, 50, 66, 70; secure, xxii, 50, 52, 57, 59, 152–53, 166; for survival, 50; working with, 163–64

attachment theory: children and, xxi, xxii, 49–54, 56–58, 152, 153; communication and, 50–52; journal prompts, 52–53; students and, 51–52, 54–60

audience, xv, 12, 36, 59, 151, 168

Austin, Diane, 68

autobiographical memory, 22

autonomic nervous system (ANS): breathing and, 11; co-regulation and, 38, 85; defined, 77; dysregulated, 32, 40, 44, 46; KATMAN technique and, 69; neuroception and, 36; PNS, xvi, xvii, xx–xxi, 8, 9, 11, 14–16, 19–21, 24, 25, 29, 32–35, 37, 40, 77–78, 80, 87, 167; PVT and, 32–35; re-regulating, 42–44; SNS, xvi, xxi, 8, 9, 11, 19, 33–35, 58, 77–78, 80–81; vagus nerve, xvii, xx–xxi, 29, 32–35, 37, 40, 197

avoidant attachment, 50, 53–56, 59, 156–57, 164–65

awareness: of attachment adaptation, 57–58; body, 23, 25–26, 34–35, 42, 80–81, 160, 165; cultivating presence and, 143–44, 148; dual, 87, 88; of exteroception, 87; of power, 83, 84; self-, 23, 25, 85–86, 115–16, 161; of transference and countertransference, 95; trauma, xxii, 146–47, 201–4

Baker, Janet, 65–66

Bartlett, Diane, 50

Becker, Diana Rose, 66

behavior, 25, 49, 58, 127, 128, 131

behavioral measures, research, 65

behavioral symptoms, trauma, 13–17

bel canto singing, 83–84, 199n6

Berntson, G., 77

bias, implicit, 178, 181–82

"Big T Trauma," 8

biological markers, PTSD, 67

BIPOC (Black and Indigenous People of Color), xix, 114

Blackness in Opera (André), 136

Black Opera (André), 136

Blacks, xix, 114, 136, 138, 183, 203, 204

"Black sound," 136

blanking out, xvi, 21, 138

blood pressure, 9, 19, 21, 23–24, 34

body, xiv, xvii, 11, 38, 104, 143, 191; awareness, 23, 25–26, 34–35, 42, 80–81, 160, 165; diversity and inclusivity, 179–83; embodiment, 80, 87–88, 115–16, 160, 195; fatphobia, 124, 173, 179; with stuck energy, xv, 10, 41–42, 79; trauma and, 8, 78; white, x, 114, 186, 189, 192; yes, no, maybe practice, 195–96

Body Perception Questionnaire (BPQ), 41, 47n24

The Body is Not an Apology (Taylor, S. R.), 80–81

The Body Keeps the Score (Van der Kolk), 4, 17, 115, 148

bodywork, 17–18, 39, 164

boredom, 17, 145

boundaries, xv, 25, 100, 102, 146–48, 155–56, 162–63

Bowlby, John, xxi, 49, 152

BPQ (Body Perception Questionnaire), 41, 47n24

Brackett, Marc, 145, 165

brain: ADHD and, 111–12; emotional, 115; healing and KATMAN technique, 69–70; mammalian, 18–19, 20, 145; neuroception, 36–37, 43, 78; neurodivergent, xix, 112, 138; neuroplasticity, 40, 42, 52, 84; parts of, 18–22, 94, 115, 131, 145, 172; reptilian, 18, 172; scans, 18, 20, 22, 23, 41; self-compassion and, 170–71; shutting down, 20–21, 22, 23; stress and, 203; trauma and, 18–19

brain, traumatic-stimuli response: amygdala goes on alert, 19–20; with changed thinking, 11; with hemispheres disconnected, 23; language and, 21–22, 50; loss of self, 23, 25; research, 23–25; thalamus shuts down, 20–21
Brazelton, T. B., 57
breathing, 13, 43, 75, 77, 78, 81, 83, 159; exercises, 31, 88, 117, 160; fundamentals, 104–5; patterns, 11, 12, 35, 36, 45–46
Broca's area, 22
brown, adrienne maree, 186, 197
Brown, Brené, 126, 127, 132, 133–34, 168
Brown, Jeb, 118–19
Brown, Michael, 4
burnout, 89, 148, 151
buzzing, 117

Cameron, Julia, 107
cancer, 13, 39, 181
CASEL (Collaborative for Academic, Social, and Emotional Learning), 161–62
CDC (Centers for Disease Control), U.S., xxii–xxiii, 4, 82, 105, 203
Center for Health Care Strategies, 93–94, 151
Center on the Developing Child, Harvard University, xviii
Centers for Disease Control (CDC), U.S., xxii–xxiii, 4, 82, 105, 203
Certificate of Clinical Competence, 98, 113
Childhood Trauma Questionnaire, 66
children, 17, 21–22, 66, 81, 131; ACEs, xxii, 3–4, 52, 90, 202–3; attachment theory and, xxi, xxii, 49–54, 56–58, 152, 153; infants, xviii, xxi, 37–38, 49–53, 56–57, 153; teens and trauma rates, xiii
choices, 82–84, 86, 100, 109, 112–14, 169, 194–95
Choral Journal (ACDA), 163–64

choral pedagogy, trauma-informed, 161, 163–64
choral singing, 201–2
Clapp, Jane, 87, 91n2, 195
clean pain, dirty and, 124, 126, 132, 150–51, 204
climate of care, 53, 106, 153
clinician, PVT and role of, 45–46
co-harmony. *See* co-regulation
collaboration, trauma-informed practice, 82, 100, 110–12
Collaborative for Academic, Social, and Emotional Learning (CASEL), 161–62
colonialism, 76, 84, 199n6, 203; decolonization, x, 83, 114, 136, 186, 194, 202
comfort, safety versus, 177
communication, 35–38, 50–52, 175–76, 178
competition, 179, 192
complaints, 31–32, 38–41, 44, 46, 211
complexity, 101, 146, 147, 150, 186
compound trauma, xxii, 5, 8
computational science, in voice and trauma, 67
conflict over speaking out (COSO), 66
consent, 83, 112, 173–78, 180, 194
consistency, 56, 114
constellations, families and systemic, 31–32
control, 59, 126, 127
Cook, Lauren A., 102, 173–74
co-regulation (co-harmony), 76, 93; absence of, 25; healthy, 59; infants with, xviii, 37–38; regulation with, 40, 52, 102, 111; singing in harmony with, 85–87
cortisol, 19, 77, 171–72
COSO (conflict over speaking out), 66
countertransference, 95
coupling, traumatic, 15–16, 37
COVID-19 pandemic, 4, 15, 69, 145, 165
cranial nerves, 33, 40. *See also* vagus nerve

210 Index

creativity, 76, 107, 108, 126, 130, 147, 164, 167
criminal behavior, 49, 58
criticism, students with, 131, 133–34, 138, 168–72
crying, xviii, 16, 56
culture, 55, 82, 107–9, 136, 151, 186, 192; gender, history and, 100, 114–20; voice, 83–84, 189, 191, 194, 199n6
curiosity, life without, 13–14
cutthroat mindset, 137
Cycle of Socialization theory, 189

Dana, Deb, 43, 85, 109, 146, 148, 149
D'Andrea, Wendy, 25
Dare to Lead (Brown, B.), 126, 127
deactivating strategy, 55
decision making, 82, 144, 162
decolonization, x, 83, 114, 136, 186, 194, 202
deloaded language, 175–77, 180, 183
Department of Health and Human Services, U.S., 203
departure stress, 166–67
depersonalization, 21
depression, 13, 30, 94, 104, 106, 115, 126, 170
developmental trauma, xv, 5–6, 8, 69. *See also* attachment theory
Diagnostic and Statistical Manual of Mental Disorders (DSM), xiii, xiv, 5, 6–7
diaphragm, 11–12, 33, 40–41, 46, 75, 78, 104. *See also* breathing
difference, honoring, 188–89, 193–94
digestive system, xx, 9, 17, 29, 34, 40–41, 102, 144
dignity, 185–93, 199n2. *See also* vocal dignity
Dijkstra, T., 67
dirty pain, 124, 126, 132, 149, 151, 204
disabilities, xix, 81, 114, 175
discovery, exploration and, 107–9
disordered breathing (hyperventilation), 75, 81

disorders, 30, 58, 96, 102–3, 159–60, 173, 181–82. *See also* posttraumatic stress disorder; voice disorders
disorganized attachment, 50, 57–60, 167
dissociation, xvi, 17, 21, 25, 37, 138, 147; defined, xvii, 16, 34, 55; self-awareness, embodiment and, 115–16
diversity, inclusivity and body, 179–83
dogs, electric shocks on, 14
dorsal shutdown, 34, 35, 148, 149
dorsal state, 36, 38, 42, 44
dorsal vagus, 33, 34, 35, 40
down-regulation, 9, 37, 167
DSM (*Diagnostic and Statistical Manual of Mental Disorders*), xiii, xiv, 5, 6–7
dual awareness, 87, 88
Durham, Megan, x
Dweck, Carol, 129, 130, 131, 132, 171
dysphonia, 65, 75, 79
dysregulation, 32, 34–35, 40–41, 44, 46, 146

ear, nose and throat (ENT) doctor, 30–31, 39, 45, 96–97, 98, 102
ears, xx, 29, 33, 40, 44, 45, 193. *See also* hearing
Eating and Weight Disorders (journal), 159
eating disorders, 102–3, 159–60, 173, 181–82
Edgar, Scott N., 161, 162
Edmondson, Amy, 106
effort, 129, 130
Eidsheim, Nina Sun, 136
electric shocks, on dogs, 14
electromyography (EMG), 23
embodiment, 80, 87–88, 115–16, 160, 195
EMDR (Eye Movement Desensitization and Reprocessing), 68–69
EMG (electromyography), 23
emotion, xiv–xv, xviii–xix, 16–17, 20, 22, 51, 85, 112, 118; CASEL, 161–62; joy, 13–14, 69, 126, 149, 186, 197–98; negative, 130, 145; neglect, xxii, 53, 66; regulation of, 50, 56–57, 111; SEL,

161–63; shame, 75, 81, 115, 126–30, 168, 200n7; suppressing, 37, 101; trauma processed with movement of, 79; vocal sounds altered by, 63, 64; Yale Center for Emotional Intelligence, 145, 162, 165
empathy, 119, 127, 148
Empowered Musician, 137
empowerment, with voice and choice, 82, 100, 112–14
endocrine system, 18, 144
energy, bodies with stuck, xv, 10, 18, 41–42, 79
ENT (ear, nose and throat) doctor, 30–31, 39, 45, 96–97, 98, 102
episodic memory, 22
ethical scope of practice, xxii; boundaries between teacher and student, xv, 25; breathing fundamentals, 104–5; language describing role of providers, 98–99; Meta-Therapy, 118–20; National Center for Voice and Speech symposium, 98–100; NATS, ASHA and VASTA joint statement, 96–97; professional ethics, 100–120; student disclosure, 102–3, 110; survey of voice teachers, 98; titles of vocal health professionals, 98–99
ethics code, 96, 100–101, 105, 110, 112–14
Eustis, Lynn, 54–55, 107–8, 124, 131–32, 149, 165
event (shock) trauma, xv, 5, 8
executive functioning, 50
exercises: breathing, 31, 117, 160; felt sense, 117; *Polyvagal Exercises for Safety and Connection*, 43; proprioception, 116; protective sphere, 168; to regulate nervous system, 43–44; resilience through, 150; self-compassion, 172–73; sound as regulating stimulus, 117; vocal dignity, 187–88, 191–93, 195–98
exploration, discovery and, 107–9
expressive skills, breathing, 105

external regulation, 25, 57
exteroception, 87
Eye Movement Desensitization and Reprocessing (EMDR), 68–69
eyes, 13–14, 33–36, 40, 51, 55, 149, 167

facial electromyography, 23
facial expressions, 22, 42–43
facial muscles, 17, 24, 40
failure, 15, 60, 126, 132, 133, 169, 190
families, 31–32, 52–53, 125, 145
fatigue, chronic, 13, 17, 75
fatphobia, 124, 173, 179
faults, survival strategies and vocal, 80
feedback, providing, 131, 132–34, 138
feeling, xvi, 13, 26, 53, 94, 145; of failure, 60, 169; felt sense, 116, 117; fully alive, 16–17; Mood Map, 165–66; numbness, xiv, xvii, 21, 75, 78–80, 88, 116, 127, 148. *See also* emotion
felt sense, 116, 117
fibromyalgia, 13, 17
Fields, Amy, 98
fight-or-flight response, xvi, xxi, 8–9, 11, 19, 33, 35, 58, 78, 81. *See also* sympathetic nervous system
Finkelstein, Zach, 179
fitness, athleticism and, 191, 200n7
fixed mindset, 129–31, 171
Floyd, George, 4
free associative singing, 68
Freely given, Reversible, Informed, Enthusiastic, Specific (FRIES), 175–76, 177
freeze (immobility) response, xvi–xviii, 20–21, 80, 87, 167; dissociation and, 16, 25, 37; fight, flight or, 8, 9, 11, 19, 78; as reinforced belief, 14–15. *See also* parasympathetic nervous system
Freud, Sigmund, xiii
FRIES (Freely given, Reversible, Informed, Enthusiastic, Specific), 175–76, 177
Fromm, Erich, 84
frontal lobes, 19–20, 22

functional abnormalities (disorders), 30
functional voice disorders, xxi, 31, 39, 63–66, 68

Gallagher, Maureen, 50
Garner, Eric, 4
gender, 82, 100, 114–20, 135–36, 164, 175
George, Carol, 52
Gilman, Marina, 98
"glissando," spectogram of, 66
globus, 41, 65
Good-Perkins, Emily, 83–84, 199n6
Gottleib, Lori, 154–55
Gray, Jeffrey, 20
grief, xiv, 63, 75
Griffin, Paul, 118, 148
grind-culture mentality, 192
Grooten, Heleen, xxi
growth mindset, 129–30, 132
guilt, 130, 147, 181, 189, 200n7

habilitation, 96, 98, 99
HAES' (Health at Every Size), 182
Haines, Staci, 77
Hapner, Edie, 98
harm, avoiding, 105
Harro, Bobbie, 186, 189
healer/therapist, voice teacher as, 84, 85
healing, xvii, 3, 17, 25–26, 52; clean pain and, 124, 126, 132, 150–51, 204; KATMAN technique and brain, 69–70
Health at Every Size (HAES)', 182
hearing, 31, 34, 41, 45, 55; ASHA, 30, 96–98, 100, 103–4, 112–13; listening, 35, 147, 154–56; mechanics of, 43–44. *See also* sounds
heart, xx, 18, 33, 40, 41; rate, 9, 13, 21, 23, 24, 77, 171; vagus nerve and, 29, 32
heart rate variability (HRV), 13, 171
Helding, Lynn, xiv, 135
Hellinger, Bert, 31
Helou, Leah B., 25, 79, 119
Helou Laboratory for Vocal Systems Anatomy and Physiology, 25

helplessness, 14–15, 21, 145, 147, 190
history: music, 149–51, 153; trauma, 12, 64, 66–68, 95, 127, 128, 151
holding, vocal, 68
homeostasis, 9, 18, 19, 144
hooks, bell, xi, 111, 186, 188
household challenges, questions, 53
HPA (hypothalamic-pituitary-adrenal) axis, 144
HRV (heart rate variability), 13, 171
human dignity, 199n2
Humane Music Education for the Common Good (Good-Perkins), 83–84, 199n6
humility, vocal dignity and, 198
humming, 117, 123, 160, 188
hydration, 30, 150
hypersensitivity, 34, 37, 44, 166
hypertonia, 36, 45
hyperventilation (disordered breathing), 75, 81
hypervigilance, 11, 13–14, 57, 78–79, 88, 116, 147
hypothalamic-pituitary-adrenal (HPA) axis, 144
hypothalamus, 18

identity, xix–xx, 175, 189, 191
illnesses, xiii, 13, 56, 80
imagination, failure of, 15
immobility response. *See* freeze response
immune system, 17, 18, 67, 144
implicit bias, 178, 181–82
imprint, 8, 10–11, 16, 38, 43, 52, 59
inclusivity, 174–83
indigenous people, x, xix, 114
inescapable shock, dogs, 14
infants: attachment theory, xxi, 49–50, 52–53, 56–57, 153; with co-regulation, xviii, 37–38; regulation and, 51, 153
Inflamed (Patel and Marya), 144–45, 203
inflammation response, 144
information, 14, 63–65
insecure attachment, 50, 66, 70
"Instagram therapy," 77

Institute of Childhood Trauma and Attachment, 21
intake session, 153
intellectual functioning, 50
Interagency Task Force for Trauma-Informed Care, 105
internal (self-) regulation, 56–57, 59
interoception, 80, 87
intrusive thoughts, 75, 81
isolation, 23, 53, 77, 120, 126–27, 135, 181
I Thought It Was Just Me (But It Isn't) (Brown, B.), 127

Janet, Pierre, xiii, 3, 16
jaw, 34, 40, 42, 44, 46
Johnson, Brittney, 183
Johnson, Kristofer, 126
journal prompts, attachment style, 52–53
joy, 13–14, 69, 126, 149, 186, 197–98
Jungian Somatics, 87, 195

Kain, Kathy, xviii, 17
Kaplan, Nancy, 52
Kardiner, Abram, xiii, 10
KATMAN technique, 69–70
Krusemark, Carol, 89–90

Laban Movement Analysis, xiv
language, 82, 119, *165*, 175–77, 180, 183; ASHA, 30, 96–98, 100, 103–4, 112–13; brain, traumatic-stimuli response and, 21–22, 50; describing role of providers, 98–99; vocal dignity and, 191–92, 200n7; written word, x, 186, 199n1; yes, no, maybe practice, 195–96. *See also* speech-language pathologist
Lanius, Ruth, 23, 25
Larman-Ivens, Freya, 134
laryngeal muscles, 39, 41, 79, 159
laryngoresponder, emotional neglect, 66
larynx, xx–xxi, 29, 33, 40, 45–46, 96, 98, 102

learning, xiv–xv, 21, 130, 135, 153, 161–63
LeDoux, Joseph, 115
Levine, Peter, ix, xiv, 3, 9, 23, 41, 42, 116–17; with incomplete survival responses, 10–11; on shock and developmental trauma, 5, 8; on trauma behavioral symptoms, 13–15
LGBTQ+ people, 136, 145
licensure laws, state, 96–97
life, 13–14, 15, 16–17, 65–66, 150, 193
limbic system (mammalian or limbic brain), 18–19, 20, 145
listening, 35, 147, 154–56
"little t trauma," 8
Lopez-Castro, Teresa, 126–27, 128–29
Lorde, Audre, 185, 186
LoVetri, Jeannette, 104
lungs, xx, 18, 33, 40

Madden, Cathy, 169
Maier, Steven, 14
Main, Mary, 50, 52, 57
mammalian brain (limbic system), 18–19, 20, 145
mantra, self-compassion, 172–73
Manual of Singing Voice Rehabilitation (Searce), xiv
"Mapping Meta-Therapy Interventions onto the Rehabilitation Treatment" (Helou), 119
Marmar, Charles R., 67
Martin, Betty, 83, 186, 194
Marya, Rupa, 144–45, 203
Maybe You Should Talk to Someone (Gottlieb), 154–55
Mazzini, Manuel Marco, 69–70
McCornack, Heather, 159–60
McLaughlin, Katie, 25
medial prefrontal cortex (MPFC), 19–20, 115
medically unexplained symptoms (MUS), 31
meditation, x, 83, 150, 151, 155, 172–73
memory, 12, 16, 20–22, 132, 143

Menakem, Resmaa, 3, 117, 124, 149, 150, 201
mental health, xv, 89, 90, 93, 105, 151; DSM, xiii, xiv, 5, 6–7; practitioners, xvii, xix, 20, 45, 111, 146, 164
mental self-care, 149
Meta-Therapy, 118–20
#metoo movement, 124
Metropolitan Opera National Competition, 179
mind, body and, 38
mindful movement, 76, 83, 116, 167, 168
mindset, 129–32, 137, 171, 192
minimizing, 147, 177
"misunderstood complaints," 31–32, 38
Montello, Louise, 69
Montello Method for Performance Wellness, 69
Monti, Elisa, 23, 67, 70, 79, 93–94, 119
Mood Map, 165–66
mouth-breathing, 11, 12, 81
"move against" behavior, 128
movement, 80, 82, 88, 99, 151, 200n7; with avoidant attachment, 164; emotional, 79; involuntary, 10, 42; mindful, 76, 83, 116, 167, 168; reduced capacity for, 78; unfinished, 41, 42. *See also* breathing
Movement for Trauma, 91n2, 144, 195
moving away and toward, behavior, 127
MPFC (medial prefrontal cortex), 19–20, 115
MUS (medically unexplained symptoms), 31
muscles, 24, 34, 36, 40, 45, 132; laryngeal, 39, 41, 79, 159; tension, xviii, 17, 33, 35, 43–44, 75, 137
music, trauma with vocal training and, xxii; feedback skills, 131, 132–34, 138; gender in voice study, 135–36; mindset, 129–32; perfectionism, 124–27, 128; race and voice, 136–38; shame, 126–29, 130; studio and, 94, 134–35

Music Education and Social–Emotional Learning (Edgar), 161
music history, 149–51, 153
The Musician's Mind (Helding), 135
music theory coursework, 130
music therapy, 68, 84, 201
mutuality, trauma-informed practice, 82, 100, 110–12
My Grandmother's Hands (Menakem), 117

National Association of Teachers of Singing (NATS), 96–97, 100–101
National Center for Voice and Speech symposium, 98–100
NATS (National Association of Teachers of Singing), 96–97, 100–101
neck, hypervigilance and, 13–14
Neff, Kristin, 169–73
neocortex, 18, 19
nervous system, xiii–xiv, xxii–xxiii, 9, 11–13, 33, 35, 43–44, 144; activation, xvi, xx, 8, 14, 15, 22, 25–26, 37, 55, 137; function, xv, xvii, xxi, 29, 146; of performers onstage, xv, xvi–xviii, 55; stuck energy in, xv, 10, 41–42, 79. *See also* autonomic nervous system
neuroception, 36–37, 43, 78
neurodivergent, xix, 112, 138
neuroplasticity, 40, 42, 52, 84
neuroscience, xiii, xiv, 169
Nix, John, 98
non-disordered voices, 64, 66–67
non-dual practice, 196–97
nose-breathing, 12, 81, 83
numbness, xiv, xvii, 21, 75, 78–80, 88, 116, 127, 148. *See also* feeling
nutrition, good, 150

onstage, nervous system of performers, xv, xvi–xviii, 55
open-ended questions, 162, 177, 180, 184n30
opera pipeline, students in, 137

organic abnormalities (voice disorders), 30
orienting response, 14, 131–32, 153
otolaryngologist. *See* ear, nose and throat doctor
Overloaded and Underprepared (Pope), 106
Ozturk, Erdinc, 55

Pace, Chelsea, 175, 180
pain, 17, 145, 172; clean, 124, 126, 132, 150–51, 204; dirty, 124, 126, 132, 149, 151, 204
Pan-American Vocology Association (PAVA), 89, 96, 100
panic attack, xvii, 16, 101–2, 125, 149
parasympathetic nervous system (PNS, rest and digest): freeze response, xvi, xvii, 8–9, 11, 14–16, 19–21, 25, 37, 78, 80, 87, 167; PNS, heart rate and, 24; SNS and, 77; vagus nerve, xvii, xx, xxi, 29, 32–35, 37, 40, 197
Patel, Raj, 144–45, 203
PAVA (Pan-American Vocology Association), 89, 96, 100
PAVA-RV (PAVA-Recognized Vocologist), 89, 100
peer support, trauma-informed practice, 82, 100, 109–10
perfectionism, xvii, 69, 124–27, 128, 192
performance anxiety, 69, 76
performer, xv, xvi–xviii, 55, 168
Permission to Feel (Brackett), 145, 165
persecution, sense of, 147
personality disorder, 58
phonation, 36, 65, 66, 81, 88
phonetogram, of vocal range, 66
phoniatrician. *See* ear, nose and throat doctor
physical self-care, 149
physical symptoms, 13, 17, 41, 127
physiological change, 12, 18
pinched voice, 39
PITS (powerlessness in the system), 66
Pleasure Activism (brown, a. m.), 197

PNS. *See* parasympathetic nervous system
Polatin, Betsy, ix
Pole, Nnamdi, 23–25
Polyvagal Exercises for Safety and Connection (Dana), 43
polyvagal theory (PVT), xvii, xx, 32, 34, 39, 46; neuroception, 36–37, 43, 78; re-regulating ANS, 42–44; social engagement system and, xxi, 29, 33, 35, 37, 40, 127; SSP case study to illustrate effect, 44–45; voice and, 35–38, 41–42
The Polyvagal Flip Chart (Dana), 43
The Polyvagal Theory in Therapy (Dana), 85
Poole Heller, Diane, 50, 52, 53, 59, 152, 153, 169
Pope, Denise, 106
Porges, Stephen, xvii, xxii, 33, 44, 127; neuroception and, 36, 78; PVT and, xx–xxi, 32–35, 41
Possibility Project, 118, 122n49
Postmodern Culture (Eidsheim), 136
Posttraumatic Growth (Tedeschi), 129
posttraumatic stress disorder (PTSD), 13, 20, 23, 69; in DSM, xiii, xiv, 5, 6–7; heart rate and, 24; shame and, 126–27; speech and, 67, 80; in veterans, 4, 16, 24–25, 67, 94
power, xvii, 50, 82, 100, 112–14, 137, 153; of co-regulation, 38; dynamics, 175, 184n30; -from-within, 189, 190; -over, 189, 190, 191, 192; in relationships, 83, 84, 192–93; -with, 189, 190, 192
powerlessness in the system (PITS), 66
The Power of Attachment (Poole Heller), 50, 153
practice: PVT in, 40; singers and trauma-informed, 81–82; vocal dignity, 187, 188, 193, 196–97; weekly log, 166; yes, no, maybe, 195–96. *See also* ethical scope of practice
practicing, talent and, 130
practitioner, autonomic state of, 42–43

praise, for talent, 129–30, 131
predator sounds, 34
predictability, clarity of expectations and, 114
presence, 53, 87–88, 143–44, 148
proprioception, 87, 116
protective sphere exercise, 168
psychogenic voice disorders, 30, 45–46, 65–66, 79
psychological illnesses, trauma and, xiii
psychological safety, 90, 106–7, 145
psychologists, xix, xx, 30; APA, 100, 105, 110, 114; with Voice and Trauma Research Group, ix
psychotherapeutic care, xxii, 64, 68, 95
psychotherapist, ix, 31, 79, 84, 95
psychotherapy, vocal, 63, 64, 68
PTSD. *See* posttraumatic stress disorder
PVT. *See* polyvagal theory

Queering Vocal Pedagogy (Sauerland), 134, 135, 163, 201

race, xix, 114, 136–38, 183, 203–4. *See also* Blacks; whites
racism, x, 4, 76, 79, 124, 138, 199n1, 203
Random Forest probability algorithm, 67
range, vocal, 66
readership, intended, xix
reading guide, xx–xxiii
reality, 16, 55
"Reel to Real" (hooks), 188
regression, 66, 174
regulation, xviii, 43, 51, 52, 102, 117, 153; down-, 9, 37, 167; dysregulation, 32, 34–35, 40–41, 44, 46, 146; of emotion, 50, 56–57, 111; external, 25, 57; internal, 56–57, 59. *See also* co-regulation
rehabilitation, xiv, 89, 98, 99–100, 119
relational self-care, 149
relationships: families, 31–32, 52–53, 125; power in, 83, 84, 192–93; teacher and student, xv, 25, 37, 54–56, 58–59, 83, 85–87, 95–96, 100, 111–12, 128, 131–35, 137–38, 145–48, 153–57, 162–63, 166
reptilian brain, 18, 172. *See also* amygdala
re-regulation, of ANS, 42–44
rescuer, 84, 85, 190, 191
research, xxi, 17, 20; additional related methods, 68–69; behavioral measures, 65; electric shocks on dogs, 14; KATMAN technique, 69–70; Montello Method for Performance Wellness, 69; music education, 136, 161; PTSD and speech / voice indicators, 67; self-report methods, 65–66; trauma and functional voice disorders, 64, 65–66; trauma history and non-disordered voices, 66–67; traumatic-stimuli response of brain, 23–25; vocal psychotherapy case studies, 63, 64, 68; voice teaching and, 70
resilience, xxii, 146, 150, 171, 188, 192, 201; growth mindset and, 130; regulation and, xviii, 59; skills, 106, 115
rest and digest. *See* parasympathetic nervous system
re-traumatization, 42, 90, 94, 162, 202
Rice, Tamir, 4
Ricks, David F., 118
Rikard, Laura, 175
risk, effort and, 129
Ristad, Eloise, 108–9
Rosen, Clark, 79
Rosenberg, Stanley, 36, 40
Royal College of Speech and Language Therapists, UK, 51
Rupert, Anna, 21, 50, 51, 52

Safe and Sound Protocol (SSP), 43–45
safe space, 83, 106, 174–78, 202
safety, 43, 82, 83, 93, 128, 164, 177; co-regulation and, 85–87; psychological, 90, 106–7, 145; trauma-informed practice, 100, 105–7

SAMHSA (Substance Abuse and Mental Health Services Administration), 90, 105
Sar, Vedat, 55
Sariya, Tanya, 126–27
Sauerland, William, 134, 135, 163–64, 201–2
Savvidou, Paola, xiv, 100
Scherer, Stefan, 67
school, mindset at, 131–32
SDOHs (social determinants of health), xxii–xxiii, 203
SE (Somatic Experiencing), ix, 10, 17, 32, 41
Searce, Leda, xiv
secure adaptation, neuroplasticity and, 52
secure attachment, xxii, 50, 52, 57, 59, 152–53, 166
SEL. *See* social emotional learning
selective serotonin reuptake inhibitors (SSRIs), 20
self, loss of, 23, 25, 59
self-actualization, teachers with, xi
self-awareness, 23, 25, 85–86, 115–16, 161
self-care, 146, 148–49
self-compassion, 169–73
Self-Compassion (Neff), 169
self-management, SEL and, 162
self-regulation (internal regulation), 56–57, 59
self-report, 65–66, 186
self-worth, 60, 191, 197
Seligman, Martin, 14
semantic memory, 22
Seminars in Speech and Language (journal), 119
SEPs (Somatic Experiencing Practitioners), ix, 17, 93
"serve and return," 51
sex, 17, 81, 175
shame, 75, 81, 115, 126–30, 168, 200n7
shock: dogs and electric, 14; shell, 38; trauma, xv, 5, 8

shutting down, 14–15, 17, 77, 101, 128, 149; blanking out, xvi, 21, 138; brain, 20–21, 22, 23; singers, 58, 190
singers, ix, xiv, xix, 15, 35–36, 44–45, 136, 190; anxious attachment in, 56–57, 166, 167; avoidant attachment in, 53–56, 164–65; body awareness, 23, 25–26, 80–81; disorganized attachment in, 58, 59–60, 167; trauma-informed practice and, 81–82. *See also* music, trauma with vocal training and
The Singer's Epiphany (Eustis), 54–55
singing, xi, xvi, xvii, 12, 68; bel canto, 83–84, 199n6; choral, 201–2; in harmony with co-regulation, 85–87; voice, xiv, xix, 35, 84, 97–99, 184n40, 186, 191, 199
singing teachers. *See* voice teachers
skin conductance, 23–24
Sky, Licia, 17
sleep, 7, 12, 13, 18, 45, 144, 145, 150
SLP. *See* speech-language pathologist
SLP Australia, 51
Snowdon, Jennifer, 11–12
SNS. *See* sympathetic nervous system
social awareness, SEL and, 162
social determinants of health (SDOHs), xxii–xxiii, 203
social emotional learning (SEL), 161–63
social engagement system, xxi, 29, 33, 35, 37, 40, 127
social workers, 43, 101, 127, 147, 168
Society for Emotion and Attachment Studies, 51
Somatic Experiencing (SE), ix, 10, 17, 32, 41
Somatic Experiencing Practitioners (SEPs), ix, 17, 93
A Soprano on Her Head (Ristad), 108–9
sounds, 16, 99, 105, 117, 136; hearing, 30–31, 34, 41, 43–45, 55, 96, 98; vocal, 14, 63, 64
sources, of trauma, 5
spectrogram, of "glissando," 66

speech, 51, 98–100, 119; PTSD and, 67, 80; talking, 40, 66, 153–54, 168; therapist, 31–32, 42, 46; trainers, 96–97. *See also* language
speech-language pathologist (SLP), ix–xxi, xiv, 21, 30, 45, 50; NATS, ASHA and VASTA on, 96–97; practitioners, xix, 51, 89–90, 96–99; vocologists, 89, 99, 100
speech pathologist. *See* speech-language pathologist
spirituality, 149, 161
SSP (Safe and Sound Protocol), 43–45
SSRIs (selective serotonin reuptake inhibitors), 20
Staging Sex (Pace), 175
Starhawk (author/activist), 189
Steele, Howard, 51
Stough, Carl, ix
Strange Situation Procedure, xxi, 49, 57
straw phonation, 88
stress, 39, 55, 79, 88, 119, 159, 171; breathing patterns, 11, 12; departure, 166–67; hormones, 12–13, 16–19, 94, 137, 153; life events with, 65–66; polyvagal theory and response to traumatic, xxi; race and, 203; teachers and, 144–46; voice disorders and, 34
students: agency, 152, 174, 178, 183, 195; attachment theory and, 51–52, 54–60; with criticism, 131, 133–34, 138, 168–72; disclosure template, 102–3, 110; with failure of imagination, 15; teacher listening to, 154–56; teacher relationship with, xv, 25, 37, 54–56, 58–59, 83, 85–87, 95–96, 100, 111–12, 128, 131–35, 137–38, 145–48, 153–57, 162–63, 166; teacher talking to, 153–54; working with anxious attachment, 166, 167. *See also* music, trauma with vocal training and; singers
studio, voice: adaptations, 165–69; consent in, 173–74; as safe space, 106; trauma in, 94, 134–35
style parameters, breathing, 104–5

sub-diaphragmatic, 40–41
Substance Abuse and Mental Health Services Administration (SAMHSA), 90, 105
"supershrink," 118
supra-diaphragmatic, 40, 41
survival, 8, 36–37, 50, 80, 127, 130, 180
survival responses, xvi, 9–11, 19, 33, 34, 59
sympathetic activation, 33, 34, 36–38, 40–42
sympathetic nervous system (SNS): fight-or-flight response, xvi, xxi, 8–9, 11, 19, 33, 35, 58, 78, 81; overactive responses, 80; PNS and, 77; PVT and, 34
sympathetic state, 11, 12, 35, 44, 45–46, 149
symptoms: behavioral, 13–17; MUS, 31; physical, 13, 17, 41, 127; with stuck energy in body, 10, 79; sudden emergence of, 8; voice disorders, 29–31
"syndromal" people, 17

talent, praise for, 129–30, 131
talking: complaints increased with, 40; COSO, 66; about shame, 168; teacher and student, 153–54
"task-based presence," attachment and, 53
Taylor, Breonna, 4
Taylor, Sonya Renee, 80–81, 186
teachers. *See* voice teachers
The Teacher's Ego (Eustis), 107, 149
teaching: self-compassion, 169–72; voice, 70, 186
Teaching the Whole Musician (Savvidou), xiv, 100
Teaching to Transgress (hooks), xi
Tedeschi, G., 129, 130
teens, trauma rates in, xiii
tenth cranial nerve. *See* vagus nerve
terminology, identity and, xix–xx
text analysis, *165*, 166

thalamus, 19, 20–21
theater, 118
therapist, 118–19
thinking: brain, trauma and changed, 11; low HRV influencing, 13; mindsets, 129–32, 137, 171, 192
Thom, Kai Cheng, 186, 198
threat orientation, 167
throat, 38, 42, 82, 168, 193; complaints, 39, 40, 41, 44, 211; cutthroat mindset, 137; ENT doctor, 30–31, 39, 45, 96–97, 98, 102; globus, 41, 65; laryngeal muscles, 39, 41, 79, 159; laryngoresponder, 66; larynx, xx–xxi, 29, 33, 40, 45–46, 96, 98, 102; social engagement and, 33
TIC. *See* trauma-informed care
tinnitus, 45
titles, vocal health professionals, 98–99
TIVC. *See* trauma-informed voice care
To Have or To Be (Fromm), 84
Tolle, Eckhart, 38
tongue, 36, 79, 80
touch, absence of, 53
Tourette's syndrome, 10–11
training: vocal, xxii, 98, 116, 134; vocologists, 99, 100. *See also* music, trauma with vocal training and
transference, 95
transparency, trauma-informed practice, 100, 107–9
trauma, xiv, 5, 8, 77–81, 90. *See also* specific topics
Trauma and Dissociation in a Cross-Cultural Perspective (Sar and Ozturk), 55
"Trauma and Stressor-Related Disorders" (DSM), xiv
trauma exposure: communication and, 50; sixteen signs of, 147–48
trauma-informed: becoming, 146–47; choral pedagogy, 161, 163–64; culture and teachers, 151; pedagogy, 101, 164, 202; six principles of, 82, 105–14

trauma-informed care (TIC), 51, 84, 89, 147; goals, 93–94, 164; Interagency Task Force for Trauma-Informed Care, 105; principles, 90, 161, 164
trauma-informed practice, professional ethics: collaboration and mutuality, 82, 100, 110–12; cultural, historical and gender issues, 100, 114–20; empowerment, voice and choice, 82, 100, 112–14; peer support, 82, 100, 109–10; safety, 100, 105–7; trustworthiness and transparency, 82, 100, 107–9
trauma-informed voice care (TIVC): case study, 81; holding space for, 159–60; McCornack on, 159–60; purpose of, 76; singing in harmony with co-regulation, 85–87; speech pathologist and, 89–90; with supportive presence embodied, 87–88; with trauma defined, 77–81; with "trauma-informed" defined, 82–85; with trauma-informed practice, 81–82
Trauma Research Foundation, 17
Trauma Stewardship (van Dernoot Lipsky), 145, 147, 149–50
Trauma Stewardship Institute, 147
traumatic coupling, 15–16, 37
The Traumatic Neuroses of War (Kardiner), xiii, 10
Tronick, Ed, 153
trustworthiness, trauma-informed practice, 82, 100, 107–9

United Kingdom (U.K.), 51
United States (U.S.): CDC, xxii–xxiii, 4, 82, 105, 203; Department of Health and Human Services, 203
University of California, Berkeley, 52
University of Michigan School of Music, Wellness Initiative, 100
upper thoracic breathing, 11, 12
U.S. *See* United States
users, voice, xix, 30, 97

vagus (tenth cranial) nerve: body-based response and, xvii; dorsal, 33, 34, 35, 40; function of, xx, 29; with heart and digestive tract, 29, 32; ventral vagal complex, xxi, 29, 33–35, 37, 40; vibration and, 197

Van der Kolk, Bessel, 4, 23, 25, 93, 105, 118, 148, 151; brain and, 18, 19, 20, 22; on creativity and fear, 126; dissociation and, 16–17; emotional regulation and, 111; fMRI scans and, 41; on helplessness, 14; peer support and, 110; on PTSD, 67, 94; secure attachment and, 152; self-awareness and, 115–16; SNS and, 9; on stress hormones, 12–13; survival mode and, 130; on trauma imprint, 10, 11

Van der Merwe, Katinka, 70

van Dernoot Lipsky, Laura, 145–50

Van der Sluis, F., 67

Van Mersbergen, Miriam, 25

Varga, Dana Lynne, 137

VASTA (Voice and Speech Trainers Association), 96–97

ventral state, 35, 37–38, 42–45, 148

ventral vagal complex: social engagement system and, xxi, 29, 33, 35, 37, 40, 127; vagus and, xxi, 29, 33–35, 37, 40

verbal abuse, 105, 137

Verdollini Abbott, Katherine, 79

vertebra, 33

veterans, xiii, 38; with incomplete survival responses, 10–11; PTSD in, 4, 16, 24–25, 67, 94

Vietnam veterans, 16, 94

violence, 67, 79, 84, 94, 199n6, 204

vocal dignity, xxii, 82, 88, 202; celebrating choices, 194–95; centering both/and, 196; defined, 187–88; denied, 188–93; honoring difference, 193–94; humility and, 198; language and, 191–92, 200n7; non-dual practice, 196–97; opening practice, 187; questions, 185–86; reflections on power, 192–93; re-sounding joy, 197–98; voicework practice, 188, 193; yes, no, maybe practice, 195–96

vocologist, 89, 96, 99, 100

voice: cues and trauma history, 67, 68; culture, 83–84, 189, 191, 194, 199n6; with empowerment and choice, 82, 100, 112–14; *Manual of Singing Voice Rehabilitation*, xiv; National Center for Voice and Speech symposium, 98–100; non-disordered, 64, 66–67; pedagogy, 80–81, 83, 86, 134, 135, 189–91, 194, 201; pinched, 39; PVT and, 35–38, 41–42; race and, 136–38; singing, xiv, xix, 35, 84, 97–99, 184n40, 186, 191, 199; study, 114, 135–36, 188; trauma and, 63–65, 67

Voice and Speech Trainers Association (VASTA), 96–97

Voice and Trauma Research Group, ix

voice care, x. *See also* trauma-informed voice care

voice disorders: case study, 39; ethical scope of practice, 97, 98–99, 119; functional, xxi, 31, 39, 63–66, 68; psychogenic, 30, 45–46, 65–66, 79; stress and, 34; symptoms, causes, next steps, 29–31. *See also* polyvagal theory

Voice Foundation, 98

voice professionals, xiv, 81, 109, 161; hypervigilance in, 13–14; knowing and knowledge of, x; NATS and, 96, 100–101; operating beyond capacity, 146–48; organizations for, 96; race, voice and, 136; social justice, service and, 202; trauma-informed, 75–76, 88, 93–94

voice teachers, ix, xx, 30, 42, 45–46, 63, 99, 161; anxious attachment in, 157; avoidant attachment in, 156–57; becoming trauma-informed, 146–47; clearing out personal music history, 149–51; with emotional skill building, 111–12; with emotional well-being as job requirement, xix; as healer/therapist, 84, 85; NATS, 96–97,

100–101; with race and voice, 136; with secure attachment skills, 152–53; with self-actualization, xi; with self-care and more, 148–49; signs of operating beyond capacity, 146–47; signs of trauma exposure response, 147–48; stress and, 144–46; student relationship with, xv, 25, 37, 54–56, 58–59, 83, 85–87, 95–96, 100, 111–12, 128, 131–35, 137–38, 145–48, 153–57, 162–63, 166; survey, 98; trauma and, xv–xvi; with trauma-informed culture, 151; with verbal abuse, 105, 137. *See also* music, trauma with vocal training and

voice teaching, 70, 186

voicework practice, vocal dignity, 188, 193

Voigt, Deborah, 179

Waking the Tiger (Levine), 5, 13–15, 116–17

Wampold, Bruce, 118–19

Wang, Wei, 79

warm-ups, vocal, 160, 164

Weber, Max, 32

Wellness Initiative, University of Michigan School of Music, 100

Wheel of Consent, 83, 194

white body supremacy, 192

whites, 3, 199n1, 202–4; bodies, x, 114, 186, 189, 192; colonialism, 83–84, 199n6

"white sound," 136

Whitten, Sarah, 143–44

WHO (World Health Organization), 203

women, 65–66, 135, 136, 186, 201

World Health Organization (WHO), 203

World War I veterans, xiii, 38

written word, x, 186, 199n1

Yale Center for Emotional Intelligence, 145, 162, 165

YAPs (young artist programs), 137

Yeatman, Nicole, 199n2

yes, no, maybe practice, 195–96

yoga, x, 43, 84, 159, 160

Yogman, M. W., 57

young artist programs (YAPs), 137

YouTube, 153

zero-sum mindset, 137

About the Editor and Contributors

Emily Jaworski Koriath (DMA, SEP, RYT-200) serves as assistant professor of voice at the University of Alabama at Birmingham. Dr. Koriath has completed all three levels of training in Somatic Experiencing, the trauma healing modalities created by psychologist Peter Levine, and works with singers to identify and move through trauma. Prior to her appointment at UAB, she taught voice and related electives at Plymouth State University in New Hampshire and spent seven years as director of choral activities at John Stark Regional High School. Emily maintains an active performing career, appearing in numerous choral-orchestral works, and onstage in recital with her husband, pianist Tad Koriath. The Koriaths explore a wide range of song repertoire, with a special focus on living, female-identifying composers, and their debut recital album *These Distances between Us* was released by Naxos Classical and named an Opera News "Critic's choice" in December 2022. In her work as a Unitarian Universalist Music Minister, she has studied anti-racist teachings, gender-affirming pedagogy, and investigated the dismantling of white supremacy culture.

Emma Lynn Abrams is a student of the Alexander Technique, and her lens as a community organizer in the realms of racial and eco-justice informs the way she approaches and invites singers into a loving, compassionate, and trauma-informed relationship with the resilient bodies that house our unique voices and stories. She holds an M.M. in vocal performance from the University of Oregon, and is a freelance soprano, composer, poet, voice teacher, and community songtender. Based in the Willamette Valley of Oregon, her work lives and breathes at the intersection of voice, power, and play.

Lauren A. Cook is a Boston-based soprano, stage director, and educator. She is on the faculty of the Holden Voice Program at Harvard University and maintains a private studio where she specializes in training crossover classical and musical theater singers. Her students have been seen in performances with various local and regional companies such as the Tanglewood Festival Chorus, Apollinaire Theatre Company, Commonwealth Shakespeare Company, and Moonbox Productions. With research interests in the topics of consent and self advocacy for singers as well the effects of the health and wellness industry on performers, she is a frequent masterclass presenter, lecturer, and writer. Lauren is also trained as a stage director and intimacy choreographer for opera, theater, and film and has directed or choreographed for MassOpera, Suffolk University, the Greater Boston Stage Company, and Lowell House Opera.

Her performance credits encompass work in opera, oratorio, musical theater, and cabaret including roles with Opera del West, Riverside Theatre Works, Anthem Theatre Company, and multiple chamber and recital music series. She holds a master of music in vocal pedagogy from the Boston Conservatory at Berklee where she studied with Christy Turnbow. She believes that singers of every level deserve evidence-based and ethical teaching and that people of all backgrounds should be represented on stage.

Megan Durham (she/her/hers) serves on the voice faculty at the University of Louisville. A trauma-informed voice care facilitator, she also works as a singing voice specialist collaborating with the Louisville Center for Voice Care. She is a certified practitioner of Transcending Sexual Trauma through Yoga (Zabie Yamasaki), Movement for Trauma (Jane Clapp), YogaVoice® (Mark Moliterno), and LifeForce Yoga® (Amy Weintraub). Megan is the education director for the Voice and Trauma Research and Connection Group, founded by Dr. Elisa Monti. She holds a master of music degree in voice pedagogy and performance from Westminster Choir College of Rider University, a bachelor of arts degree in music from the University of Richmond, and studied singing voice habilitation with Dr. Karen Wicklund. She has previously served on the voice faculties of DeSales University, Lehigh University, Moravian College, and Muhlenberg College.

Heleen Grooten's speech pathology career began in 1979, when she opened her practice specializing in voice and breathing therapy. She immediately immersed herself in new visions of the field of breathing and systemic therapy and has gone on to train colleagues in these fields. Heleen was the project leader of a Dutch research team focused on systemic backgrounds of medically unexplained complaints. This interest in medically unexplained symptoms led to further study in body-oriented trauma therapy. Through this work, she met Dr. Stephen Porges and studied the polyvagal theory. At Porges's request, Grooten has conducted research on the efficacy of the Safe and Sound Protocol, a methodology aimed at calming the autonomic nervous system. With Elisa Monti and Megan Durham, Heleen was a cofounder of the Voice and Trauma Research and Connection Group (voiceandtrauma.com). Her current work consists of treating people with functional voice and throat complaints with trauma in the background, and she gives lectures and workshops (inter)nationally on polyvagal theory.

Dr. Elisa Monti is a psychologist with a PhD from the New School for Social Research. Her concentration is the relationship between psychological trauma and voice. Her mission is to contribute to further our understanding of this relationship. Elisa is a certified Performance Wellness therapist trained in the Montello Method for Performance Wellness and is certified in Vocal Psychotherapy (trained by Dr. Diane Austin). Elisa collaborates with numerous scholars and scientists, including the Helou Laboratory at the University of Pittsburgh and New York Speech Pathology. She is also the president and cofounder of the Voice and Trauma Research and Connection Group. Elisa has been the recipient of honors and awards, including the Audio-Visual Media Award (2017) from the International Society for the Study of Trauma and Dissociation.

www.ingramcontent.com/pod-product-compliance
Lightning Source LLC
Chambersburg PA
CBHW022011300426
44117CB00005B/133